# Wasting Away

## The Crisis of Malnutrition in India

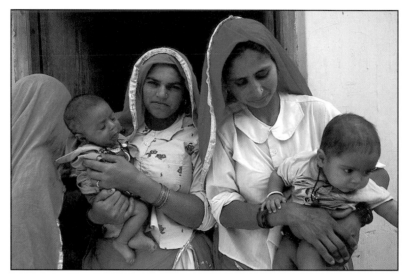
*Two mothers with their healthy children, Sultanpur, Hayana*

# DIRECTIONS IN DEVELOPMENT

# Wasting Away

## The Crisis of Malnutrition in India

Anthony R. Measham
Meera Chatterjee

The World Bank
Washington, D.C.

Cover photograph: A mother with two mildly malnourished children in a Gujarati village, by Meera Chatterjee. All interior photographs by Meera Chatterjee.

**Library of Congress Cataloging-in-Publication Data**

Measham, Anthony R.
    Wasting away : the crisis of malnutrition in India / Anthony R. Measham,
Meera Chatterjee.
        p.   cm. — (Directions in development)
      ISBN 0-8213-4435-8
      1. Malnutrition—India.   I. Chatterjee, Meera.   II. Title.
    III. Series: Directions in development (Washington, D.C.)
    RA645.N87M425    1999
    362.1'9639'00954—dc21                  99-28089
                                               CIP

# Contents

# Foreword

Fasten your seat belts. This, for some readers, is going to be a bumpy ride. In fact, before you delve further into this important new study, you should be aware that it is a most unusual publication for the World Bank. During a quarter century of association with the Bank, I have never come upon anything quite like it. The double entendre in the book's title itself is a clue to what's to come.

*Wasting Away* describes not only the physical wasting wrought by malnutrition, but the wasting of vast financial resources ostensibly being made available to address the problem. It includes at the same time both a powerful analysis of what the authors call the "silent emergency of malnutrition," and an unusually frank indictment of how it is being addressed.

Authors Anthony Measham and Meera Chatterjee, both thoroughly immersed in nutrition operations, are deeply committed to the betterment of nutrition in India. But clearly both also are deeply disappointed by the decline, compared with earlier periods, of the country's ability to effectively address the problem. Performance in nutrition indicators lag, they report, while progress on all other major social indicators has advanced impressively.

The report concludes that the implementation of India's nutrition policies has been inadequate and that India's institutional capacity in nutrition is weak. Community ownership and management of the nationwide nutrition program (ICDS) is virtually nonexistent. The program's quality of services is low, and its effect remains unknown, since no monitoring and evaluation system exists that can reliably gauge its impact on its primary objectives. Other ongoing programs, although apparently well conceived, reveal weak implementation, particularly with regard to ensuring the access of the poor; and there are virtually no synergies between them. Is it any surprise that India is unlikely to meet its stated national nutrition goals for the year 2000?

What can be done about it? The authors write a creative and useful prescription—and issue a powerful challenge. Additional resources are necessary to turn the situation around. "India is not spending enough on direct nutrition programs by any standard," the authors conclude. Sri Lanka, for instance, spends proportionately five times more—with markedly greater impact on nutrition. Other countries in the region also show better results. The cost of additional needs for activities that could make a difference is calculated at about $80 million a year for 10 years. But many of the prescribed actions involve relatively little additional

cost. There also is scope to improve dramatically the returns on existing investments.

In short, the study challenges the government to stop wasting financial resources on a number of unfruitful programs and to use what
is available more efficiently. An effective, high-quality ICDS program,
plus a well-targeted and less corrupt Public Distribution System, would
go a long way toward improving the situation, conclude the authors,
especially if the government phases out ineffective programs at the
same time.

The necessary additional $80 million a year is not a trivial amount.
But considering that the cost of malnutrition in lost productivity, illness and death is at least $10 billion a year, this is a bargain that should
not be passed up.

The authors make a strong case that India's development will be seriously impeded if the problem is not dealt with expeditiously. Malnutrition is not just a consequence of slow economic growth but a cause of
it, they say. Overcoming malnutrition, they contend, is a precondition
of growth. It would be a tragedy if India's significant strides in development in other areas are impeded by such an obstacle, especially since
the government earlier demonstrated in the states of Kerala and Tamil
Nadu that making a consequential dent in malnutrition is possible. In
fact, successful Indian programs have been looked upon as models for
community-based nutrition programs by other countries. But some of
these other countries are now surpassing their mentor, both in expanding the scale and improving upon that pioneering work. To this long-
time observer of India, it is disheartening to see the reduced condition
of India's place in international nutrition today, compared to the years
when India's nutritional scientists and institutions were among the best
in the world, and when India was looked to both for fresh ideas and as
an example of what can be achieved when a government takes the nutrition problem seriously.

This study implicitly poses a challenge to the World Bank, which has
invested three quarters of a billion dollars in the improvement of nutrition in India  more, by far, than in any other country. Should it con-
tinue to make sizable funds available to those governments with
inadequate commitment to nutritional improvement without ensuring
that the investments yield the intended results? And what can it do
differently to help bring about more positive outcomes? Although some
World Bank-assisted efforts in India have had dramatically positive
results, why have the lessons of such experience not been adopted more
broadly there?

It will be interesting to see if readers of this significant study accept
it in the constructive spirit in which it is intended. It also will be inter-

esting to look back some years from now to see what effect, if any, it may have had.

Alan Berg

Before his retirement as Senior Nutrition Adviser for the World Bank, Alan Berg lived in India and worked for four years to improve nutrition among the population. Mr. Berg has had an ongoing involvement with the subject there for more than three decades. His book, *The Nutrition Factor: It's Role in National Development*, draws significantly on his experience in India.

# Acknowledgments

This report was written by Anthony Measham (Task Leader and Adviser, Health, Nutrition and Population (HNP) Unit) and Meera Chatterjee (Co-Task Leader and Senior Social Development Specialist), with assistance from James Levinson (Consultant), Meera Priyadarshi (Nutrition Specialist), Krishna Rao (Research Associate), and Nira Singh (Office Administrator). Professors James Levinson and Rokkam Radhakrishna contributed background papers that were invaluable in preparing the report. Alan Berg, Kalanidhi Subbarao, and Olivia Yambi served as peer reviewers. The collaboration of the Department of Women and Child Development, Government of India, is gratefully acknowledged.

The draft of this report was discussed in a workshop on June 17, 1998, in New Delhi, chaired by the Department of Women and Child Development, Ministry of Human Resource Development, Government of India. The authors acknowledge with appreciation the helpful comments of the 50 participants in that workshop , as well as comments received from many other colleagues in India, the World Bank, and elsewhere, who are too numerous to name. We wish to acknowledge especially comments from Deepak Ahluwalia, Alan Berg, Kalyan Bagchi, Benoit Blarel, R. Devadas, Shanti Ghosh, Stuart Gillespie, C. Gopalan, Tara Gopaldas, Ward Heneveld, Peter Heywood, James Levinson, John Mason, Judith McGuire, Mildred McLachlan, G.V. Ramana, Suneeta Singh, Richard Skolnik, Kalanidhi Subbarao, Dina Umali-Deininger, UNICEF colleagues, and John Williamson.

The report was written under the direction of Richard Skolnik, Sector Manager, the HNP Unit, South Asia Region, and Edward Lim, Country Director, India.

# Acronyms and Abbreviations

| | |
|---|---|
| ANM | Auxiliary nurse midwife |
| AWC | *Anganwadi* center |
| AWW | *Anganwadi* worker |
| BPL | Below poverty line |
| CFTRI | Central Food Technology Research Institute |
| CHC | Community Health Center |
| CSS | Centrally sponsored scheme |
| DPEP | District Primary Education Program |
| DWCRA | Development of Women and Children in Rural Areas |
| ECD | Early childhood development |
| EPI | Expanded Program of Immunization |
| FCI | Food Corporation of India |
| GDP | Gross domestic product |
| GNP | Gross national product |
| GOI | Government of India |
| ICDS | Integrated Child Development Services |
| IDD | Iodine deficiency disorders |
| IIPS | International Institute of Population Sciences |
| IMR | Infant mortality rate |
| IRDP | Integrated Rural Development Program |
| JRY | *Jawahar Rozgar Yojana* |
| MCH | Maternal and child health |
| MIS | Management Information System |
| MOHFW | Ministry of Health and Family Welfare |
| NCAER | National Council of Applied Economic Research |
| NFHS | National Family Health Survey |
| NIN | National Institute of Nutrition |
| NIPCCD | National Institute of Public Cooperation and Child Development |
| NMMP | National Mid-day Meals Program |
| NNC | National Nutrition Council |
| NNMB | National Nutrition Monitoring Bureau |
| NPAN | National Plan of Action for Nutrition |
| NREP | National Rural Employment Program |
| NRY | *Nehru Rozgar Yojana* |
| NSS | National Sample Survey |
| PDS | Public Distribution System |

PEM        Protein-energy malnutrition
PHC        Primary Health Center
RCH        Reproductive and Child Health
RLEGP      Rural Landless Employment Guarantee Program
SDP        State domestic product
TINP       Tamil Nadu Integrated Nutrition Project
TPDS       Targeted Public Distribution System
UIP        Universal Immunization Program
ZP         *Zilla Parishad*

# Executive Summary

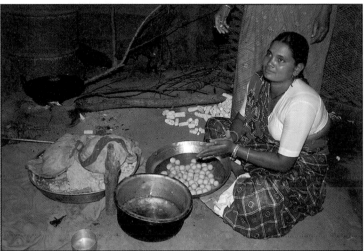

*Preparing supplementary food at an ICDS* Anganwadi *in Gujarat*

Despite India's substantial progress in human development since its independence in 1947, more that half of its children under four years of age are moderately or severely malnourished, 30 percent of newborns are significantly underweight, and 60 percent of Indian women are anemic. Malnutrition is now seriously retarding improvements in human development and further reduction of childhood mortality.

This report results from the continuing Government of India–World Bank (GOI/Bank) collaboration on the issue of nutrition, which began in 1980. As part of that collaboration, this report aims to review the effectiveness, efficiency, and impact of public spending on nutrition in India and to suggest how these might be enhanced. Several completed and ongoing GOI/ Bank studies—on poverty, rural development, and food-grain marketing— complement this report. A synthesis report on food security and nutrition also will be prepared in 1999.

India no longer faces the famine and epidemics that made life expectancy barely more than 30 years at the time of its independence. Despite progress in food production, disease control, and economic and social development, India accounts for 40 percent of the world's malnourished children while containing less than 20 percent of the global child population. Malnutrition varies widely across regions, states, age, gender, and social groups, being worst in children under two, in the large northern states, and among women, tribal populations, and scheduled castes. Fortunately, the most severe form of malnutrition has declined by one-half in the past 25 years.

Malnutrition among young children and pregnant women—the most vulnerable groups—has three main causes: inadequate food intakes; disease, including common diarrhea; and deleterious caring practices, such as delayed complementary feeding. Poverty and gender inequity are among the most important factors responsible for the high level of undernourishment. Malnourished children are unlikely to reach their physical or mental potential. The cost of malnutrition to India's gross domestic product (GDP) was estimated to be at least US$10 billion in 1996 (all dollar amounts are current U.S. dollars; a billion is 1,000 million).

Since its independence India has taken the problem of malnutrition seriously—more so than many other countries—and has developed appropriate policies and mounted major programs to address it. These include the Public Distribution System (PDS), the Integrated Child Development Services (ICDS) program, the National Mid-day Meals Program (NMMP), and several employment schemes providing food for work. Overall, however, these policies and programs have had relatively limited impact on nutrition among the poor because of major problems in effective targeting, implementation, and coverage. The PDS, for example, fails to reach the majority of the poor despite absorbing 0.5 percent of GDP. This problem was acknowledged recently in the PDS's reformulation as the Targeted PDS (TPDS). Similarly, the ICDS program covers less than one-half of the target population with poor quality services after more than 20 years of operation.

National nutrition goals set for the year 2000 may not be achieved even by 2010. India spends much less than necessary to deal with its malnutrition problem. Spending on direct nutritional programs, mainly the ICDS, the NMMP, and the micronutrient programs, now amounts to 0.19 percent of gross national product (GNP). Sri Lanka, which successfully dealt with malnutrition in the 1980s, spent about 1 percent of GNP on direct nutritional programs while simultaneously improving health services, education for females, and antipoverty measures. Spending by Indian states varies dramatically and most do not allocate resources commensurate with their levels of poverty or malnutrition.

If India is to succeed in dealing with malnutrition, the first essential requirement is a higher level of sustained political commitment. This will

require a policy and implementation structure that will actively lead, monitor, and sustain national, state, and local action in many sectors, including
agriculture, industry, and water and sanitation, in addition to implementation of the programs already mentioned. Success will also require a major effort to better target nutritional programs and substantially increase
their quality and impact. Decentralization of program implementation and
major involvement of *panchayati raj* institutions, where they work on be-
half of the poor, will be crucial. An annual review in a highly visible national forum of progress made in the nation's nutritional goals also will be
imperative to maintain the momentum.

Households below the poverty line (BPL)[1] must be reached by all of
the nutritional programs in order to achieve a major impact: the employment schemes and the TPDS to assure adequate income and food availability; the ICDS to meet the nutrition and health care needs of young
children and pregnant women; and the NMMP to provide school-age children with the incentive and nutritional support to learn. This report rec-
ommends the following priority actions for each of the major nutrition
efforts:

## Integrated Child Development Services Program

• Reach 6–24-month-old children as well as pregnant women, especially
those living in hamlets, either by hiring a second worker or by separating
the preschool education component for 3–6-year-olds from the rest of the
program.

• Enhance quality markedly through better training, supervision, and
community ownership.

• Establish a reliable monitoring and evaluation system as soon as possible.

• Freeze further expansion until quality and impact are improved mea-
surably and meet substantially higher standards in current program areas, which should be achievable with sincere efforts within three to five
years.

## Public Distribution System

• Target the PDS effectively to the poor, directing the entire food subsidy
at the population below the poverty line.

• Carefully monitor the TPDS program to ensure that it reaches the poor.

• Reallocate 10 percent of the PDS budget to the ICDS program, starting in 2002 if the ICDS's service quality has improved sufficiently by then to finance the ICDS expansion to cover all those in need.

## National Mid-Day Meals Program

• Target by area, using low educational attainment and poverty criteria.

• Target preschool as well as primary school children in areas not covered by ICDS.

• Provide a mid-morning snack rather than take-home rations or a mid-day meal.

## Health Sector

• Invest heavily in upgrading the nutritional skills of all health workers, including doctors, e.g., in managing moderate and severe malnutrition, counseling parents of sick children, and assuring iron-folate supplementation for all pregnant women.

• Improve collaboration between the *anganwadi* worker and the auxiliary nurse-midwife, particularly to achieve full coverage of 6–24-month-old children and pregnant women.

## Rebuild Institutional Capacity

• Rebuild India's eroded capacity for nutritional action, training, research, and advocacy by making key nutrition institutions autonomous and by investing in nutrition institutions, including the NIN, NIPCCD, CFTRI, colleges of home science, and nutrition-related departments in medical colleges.

• Advocate wide attention to nutrition, for example, among politicians, those concerned with the improvement of Indian women's status, and national data collecting agencies.

Lost productivity, illness, and death caused by malnutrition cost India at least US$10 billion every year. The cost of the actions proposed above would be relatively small, about US$80 million per year for 10 years. The cost of expanding an improved ICDS program could be financed by reallocating about 10 percent of the PDS budget after 2002. Nothing less than these measures will deal with the crisis of malnutrition in India.

# Chapter 1

# Why Review Nutrition?

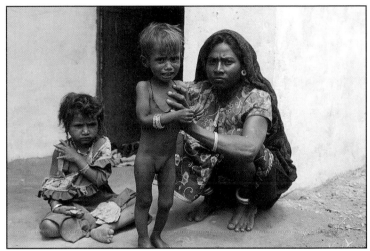

*A severely malnourished child in a tribal family in Panchmahals, Gujarat*

Since 1947, India has made substantial progress in human development. In 50 years, life expectancy has doubled, mortality has fallen by more than one-half, and fertility has declined by more than two-fifths. Poverty levels have been reduced by about two-fifths, from over 50 percent in the 1950s to 35 percent in the 1990s. Nutritional status has also improved. Famine no longer stalks the land, the country has become self-sufficient in food— one of the world's great achievements in development—and the extreme ravages of malnutrition, such as kwashiorkor and marasmus, are now relatively rare. Yet more than half of Indian children under five years of age are moderately or severely malnourished, 30 percent of newborns are significantly underweight, and 60 percent of Indian women are anemic. These manifestations of malnutrition are unacceptable. They reflect the neglect of children and women and their high risk of illness and death. They end in failure to achieve full physical and mental potential, lower productivity, and blighted lives.

Improvements in nutritional status have not kept pace with progress in other areas of human development. There are several reasons for this situation. First, nutritional status is closely linked to poverty and gender inequity, both of which remain grave problems in India. Second, most malnutrition[2] is less visible than other forms of human suffering and commands less urgent attention. Third, improvements in nutrition require a relatively complicated and interrelated set of actions for which substantial capacity, coordination, and commitment are essential. Malnutrition is now seriously retarding improvements in human development more broadly. For example, growing evidence suggests that reductions in infant and child mortality become increasingly hard to achieve. During 1991–95, the infant mortality rate (IMR) declined by 7.5 percent, compared with 17 percent in the period 1986–90. Malnutrition in India is presently a silent emergency demanding greater priority than ever before.

## The Reasons for a Review

Beginning in 1980, with the Tamil Nadu Integrated Nutrition Project (TINP), the Government of India and the World Bank have cooperated to improve nutrition in India. Since then, the Bank has financed a second phase of TINP as well as four projects in support of the ICDS program in nine states. Bank assistance to India has totaled US$753 million, equivalent to more than one-quarter of Bank assistance to improve nutrition worldwide over the past 18 years. Within India, Bank assistance to Central Government expenditures on the ICDS program has doubled, from about 15 to 30 percent between 1991 and 1998. No other donor, except UNICEF, provides sizable support to the ICDS program, but CARE and the World Food Programme give commodity assistance. In 1997 the GOI and the Bank agreed to conduct a collaborative review of nutrition to inform further joint action in this area. Accordingly, the objective of the analysis and dialogue summarized in this report is to review the effectiveness, efficiency, and impact of public spending on nutrition programs in India, and to identify how these could be enhanced.

The GOI and the Bank have collaborated and are currently collaborating on a series of related analyses, including "India: Achievements and Challenges in Reducing Poverty,"[3] "Reducing Poverty in India: Options for More Effective Public Services,"[4] "Rural Development: Options for a Growth, Poverty Oriented Fiscal Adjustment Strategy,"[5] "India–Foodgrain Marketing Policies: Reforming to Meet Food Security Needs,"[6] and a planned "Summary Report on Food Security and Nutrition in India." This report complements these other studies.

The report will focus on selected major issues that have emerged from ongoing dialogue between the Bank and the GOI and nongovernmental counterparts, including a National Nutrition Workshop on September 2–3, 1998, and a GOI/Bank workshop on June 17, 1998. It draws extensively on background papers by Professors James Levinson and Rokkam Radhakrishna and the large body of literature on nutrition programs in India. Chapter 2 describes the changing face of nutrition in India and the current situation, causes, and consequences of malnutrition. Chapter 3 summarizes plans and programs implemented since independence and discusses the extent to which the poor are being reached by these efforts and their effectiveness and efficiency, as well as public spending on nutrition. Chapter 4 sets forth conclusions and recommendations for action in four areas:

- Building India's commitment and institutional capacity to combat malnutrition
- Enhancing substantially the quality and impact of the ICDS program
- Strengthening the health sector's commitment to nutrition
- Improving food security at the community and household level

# Chapter 2

# Malnutrition in India: A Changing Picture

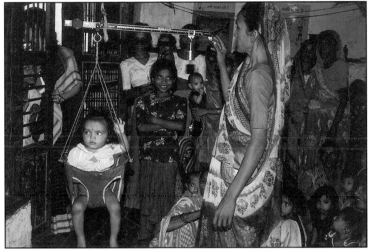

*Growth monitoring to measure children's nutritional status in the ICDS program in Gujarat*

Prior to 1947, national food shortages and a very high burden of disease, often resulting in famine and epidemics, kept life expectancy in India barely over 30 years. Low agricultural production, undeveloped transportation systems, discrimination based on gender and caste, and woefully inadequate water and sanitation made life short and harsh for the majority of Indians. Extreme forms of protein-energy malnutrition (PEM) and deficiencies of micronutrients (vitamins A, B, C, and D, iodine and iron) were commonly seen.

Since 1947, India has made great strides in food production and distribution and in the control of infections, which have significantly changed the nutritional picture. Several vitamin deficiency diseases have abated or greatly diminished. By the mid-1960s, nutritionists and medical practitioners had begun to use growth retardation in children as the main yardstick of malnutrition, a more subtle measure than the frank signs of malnutrition that were visible earlier. Degrees of underweight for age were classified as "severe," "moderate," or "mild." Today these are the main indicators of malnutrition among individuals (children); they are also a marker of households where food, health, or caring practices are inadequate.

## The Current Situation

*The Silent Emergency.* India accounts for less than 20 percent of the world's child population, but it has 40 percent of the malnourished children. PEM is the most widely prevalent form of malnutrition among children: over one-half (53 percent) of those under four years old have the moderate and severe forms (International Institute for Population Sciences [IIPS], 1995).[7] India, and South Asia as a whole, have higher rates of malnutrition than any other region of the world, including Sub-Saharan Africa. Among large countries, India ranks second only to Bangladesh in the proportion of young children affected by malnutrition. In addition, iron deficiency anemia is rampant among children and women, especially pregnant women. A nationwide survey found that 87 percent of pregnant women were anemic (Indian Council of Medical Research, 1989).[8] Vitamin A and iodine deficiency diseases are the other serious problems, concentrated in specific areas. These micronutrient deficiencies seriously affect physical and mental performance in individuals and increase the country's burden of disease.

Malnutrition varies widely across regions, states, age, gender and social groups, being worst in children under two, in the populous northern states, in rural areas, and among women, tribal populations, and scheduled castes. For example, in Kerala, 29 percent of children under four years of age are moderately or severely underweight, while the corresponding figures for Bihar and Uttar Pradesh are 63 and 59 percent, respectively (IIPS, 1995).[9]

Evidence from many sources demonstrates that malnutrition, while still unacceptably high, has declined substantially in the past two decades. For example, National Nutrition Monitoring Bureau (NNMB) data from eight states show that severe protein-energy malnutrition declined from 15 percent in 1975 to less than 7 percent in 1996 among 1–5-year-old children, and severe and moderate malnutrition combined among these children declined from about 63 to 49 percent in the same period. The National Family Health Survey of 1992–93 provides a comparable figure of 53 percent severe and moderate malnutrition among 0–4-year-olds in the country as a whole. Similar progress is evident in micronutrient malnutrition.

## Causes and Consequences of Malnutrition in India

Malnutrition is most serious among the most physically vulnerable—young children, particularly those under two, and pregnant women. Very young children require much more food per kilogram of body weight than adults, a fact that is inadequately understood. The vulnerability of pregnant women is also related to their nutritional status during adolescence.

Malnutrition results from a combination of three key factors: inadequate food intake; illness; and deleterious caring practices. Underlying these are household food insecurity, inadequate preventive and curative health services, and insufficient knowledge of proper care. In India, household food insecurity stems from inadequate employment and incomes; seasonal migration, especially among tribal populations; relatively high food prices; geographic and seasonal maldistribution of food; poor social organization; and large family size. The country still has a high incidence of disease, especially preventable communicable diseases, and maintains inadequate health services. In addition, caring practices in the home—including feeding, hygiene, home-based health care, use of available health services, and psychosocial stimulation of children—are inadequate, due substantially to the lack of education, knowledge, skills, and time among families, especially mothers. These problems are rooted in the sociocultural and economic processes that determine access to and control over resources, including information, education, assets, income, time, and even how resource-allocation decisions are made in society.

A major determinant of protein energy malnutrition (PEM) is household caloric inadequacy. According to the 1993–94 round of the National Sample Survey (NSS), the most recent major round available, about 80 percent of the rural population and 70 percent of the urban population had caloric intakes below the 2,400 calories per adult recommended for rural areas and 2,100 calories recommended for urban areas. In 1993–94 the poorest 30 percent of India's population (about 300 million people) consumed, on average, fewer than 1,700 calories per day. The poorest 10 percent consumed less than 1,300 calories per day (Shariff and Mallick, 1998).[10] At lower levels of caloric intake, people simply do not survive for long.

While poverty largely explains the high level of malnutrition in India, additional factors are responsible for the concentration of the problem among women and children. Foremost among these is the low status of women in Indian society, which results in women and girls getting less than their fair share of household food and health care. Adult women comprise one-third of India's labor force and are usually engaged in heavy manual tasks that place additional caloric demands on them. Women's heavy burden of child-bearing adds to the problem: India's total fertility rate is still 3.5 children per woman. Poor eating habits during pregnancy itself, such as "eating down" in fear of a difficult delivery caused by a large baby, and proscriptions against certain foods are widespread even among urban dwellers. The majority of Indian women are not reached by education, or even nutrition and health information of practical relevance, which could help to rectify some of these problems. Inadequate diets among the poor, skewed intrahousehold distribution of food, and inadequate caring practices result in the high rate of anemia and inadequate weight gain among pregnant women, and low birth weight among their infants.

Lack of information and education among women also underlies child malnourishment. Low birthweight babies will most likely remain on a low-growth trajectory, susceptible to malnutrition, disease, and death. While breast-feeding fortunately remains a prevalent practice in India, exclusive breast-feeding is rare, and the use of inappropriate liquids such as "sugar-water" conveys infections that cause growth faltering to begin soon after birth. In addition, the age of introduction of nutritious complementary foods is unacceptably high. The average Indian child in a poor family still receives little more than breast milk and unhygienic fluids up to the age of nine months, instead of beginning on other foods around five months. Thereafter, although semisolid foods may be given, young children are fed an insufficient number of times per day, and get a diet of inadequate quality. Coupled with the heavy load of infections and the lack of basic health care, children fall into low-growth paths and often succumb to one of the common illnesses—diarrhea or acute respiratory tract infections being among the commonest causes of death.

Malnutrition is directly or indirectly responsible for more than half of the deaths of children under five years of age worldwide. While India has successfully brought down infant mortality from 146 per 1,000 live births in 1951 to 72 in 1996, most of the children who survive are malnourished (GOI, 1998).[11] Indeed, widespread malnutrition among children and mothers is a major barrier to further reduction in mortality rates, including those among pregnant women. India's maternal mortality ratio (MMR) of 420 per 100,000 live births is unacceptably high (IIPS, 1995).[12] The country accounts for approximately one-quarter of all maternal deaths worldwide.

High levels of anemia, low pregnancy weight gain, repeated acute infections, major chronic diseases, such as tuberculosis, and inappropriate management of deliveries are important determinants of maternal and infant deaths. A large proportion of adult Indian women are at high risk of maternal mortality because their low prepregnancy height or weight may cause obstetrical difficulties. Moreover, a vicious intergenerational cycle commences when a malnourished or ill mother gives birth to a low birthweight female child: she remains small in stature and pelvic size due to further malnourishment, and produces malnourished children in the next generation.

Malnourishment can also significantly lower cognitive development and learning achievement during the preschool and school years, and subsequently result in low worker productivity. Nutritional anemia is implicated in low physical and mental performance and is exacerbated by common worm infestations. Malnutrition not only blights the lives of individuals and families, but also reduces the returns on investment in education and acts as a major barrier to social and economic progress. Malnutrition reduced India's GDP by between 3 and 9 percent in 1996, or by approximately US$10 billion–$28 billion (Administrative Staff College of India (ASCI), 1997).[13] The higher figure is greater than the sum of India's current public expenditures on nutrition, health, and education combined.

While mortality has declined by one-half and fertility by two-fifths, malnutrition has only come down by about one-fifth in the last 40 years. The inescapable conclusion is that further progress in human development in India will be difficult to achieve unless malnutrition is tackled with greater vigor and more rapid improvement in the future than in the past.

Chapter 3

# The Response: What India Has Done to Improve Nutrition

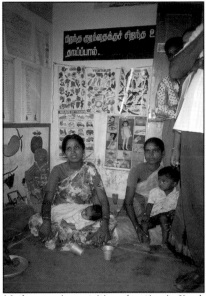

*Mothers receive nutrition education in Kerala*

Following a long history of nutritional efforts, India established in 1993 National Nutrition Goals for the year 2000. The most important of these are the following:

* Reduce by one-half severe and moderate malnutrition among young children.
* Reduce below 10 percent the incidence of low birth weight.
* Eliminate blindness due to vitamin A deficiency.
* Reduce to 25 percent iron deficiency anemia in pregnant women.
* Reduce to 10 percent iodine deficiency disorders, through salt iodization.
* Produce 250 million metric tons of food grains.
* Improve household food security through poverty alleviation programs.

As the year 2000 approaches, however, it is clear that none of these goals is likely to be met: the rates of malnutrition and poverty remain far greater than planned, and food-grain production is below expected levels. What has gone wrong? This chapter examines what India has done since its independence to address the malnutrition problem, and why these efforts have failed to produce the expected results.

Since the 1950s, India has, relative to most other countries, taken its malnutrition problem seriously in policy-making and planning, and mounted important programs to address it. In the first two Five-Year Plans (1952–61), nutritional efforts consisted of public health measures to prevent nutritional deficiencies, maternal and child feeding, and school feeding programs, and development of the food and vitamin industries. During the 1960s, increased food production was the advocated solution, and India's achievement of self-sufficiency in food grains as a result of the Green Revolution in the 1970s is well known.

These approaches formed the core of integrated efforts to address malnutrition, based on an understanding of its multiple causes. The first national nutritional scheme, the Applied Nutrition Programme, introduced in 1961, combined a demonstration approach to increasing food production at the village level ("kitchen gardening" or "nutrition extension") with an important new element: nutrition education. Recognition that malnutrition persisted despite the achievement of national self-sufficiency in food led to increased emphasis on supplementary feeding programs, and the health sector launched national prophylactic schemes against anemia and nutritional blindness (vitamin A deficiency), targeted to women and children.

In the Fifth Plan (1974–79), India introduced the Integrated Child Development Services (ICDS) program, which combined nutrition and health education, supplementary feeding, maternal and child health services, and preschool education. This effort constitutes India's longest-running nutritional program and the world's largest. It expanded rapidly from 100 blocks at the end of the Fifth Plan period to 1,000 blocks in the Sixth Plan (1980–85), to about 2,000 in the Seventh Plan (1985–90), and to more than 4,000 or 70 percent of the 5,738 development blocks in the country during the Eighth Plan period (1992–97). Although the Government of India proposed to universalize the program, i.e., to cover all rural areas and urban slums in the country, during the Eighth Plan period, it ran short of resources, leaving this goal to be achieved, possibly during the Ninth Plan (1997–2002).

The 1980s also saw the extension of the Public Distribution System (PDS), and food-for-work gained importance as a household nutrition support measure through the National Rural Employment Program (NREP). Various state-level schemes aimed at alleviating poverty were also developed. The well-known "two-rupee rice scheme" provided a large food subsidy, which has subsequently been reduced, to the people of Andhra Pradesh, and inspired modifications of the PDS. A first revision, the Revamped PDS, focused on providing subsidized food to "all people in poor areas," while the Targeted PDS (TPDS), which began in 1997, aims to provide food for "poor people in all areas."[14]

Maharashtra's successful Employment Guarantee Scheme ultimately encouraged the revamping of centrally sponsored employment programs such as the Rural Landless Employment Guarantee Programme (RLEGP), which was combined with the NREP to form the (rural) *Jawahar Rozgar Yojana* (JRY) in 1989 (and urban *Nehru Rozgar Yojana* in 1990). These schemes provide direct nutritional support to participating households by paying part of the workers' wages in the form of foodgrain (1 kilogram per person-day worked). This approach was carried forward by the Employment Assurance Scheme (EAS), and the recent TPDS also makes provision for grain payments to workers from households below the poverty line.

In Tamil Nadu, the chief minister's Noon Meal Program, begun in 1982, feeds large numbers of preschool and school children daily. The apparent success of this scheme, the presence of school meal programs in several other states, and the availability of large buffer stocks led to the expansion of midday meals as a national program in 1995. Over time, the micronutrient supplementation programs run by the Ministry of Health and Family Welfare, namely, the National Anemia Prophylaxis Programme, vitamin A distribution, and National Iodine Deficiency Disorders Control Programme have also expanded nationwide.

## Nutrition Policy for the Twenty-First Century

India formulated its National Nutrition Policy in 1993 (GOI, 1993).[15] The policy stresses the importance of direct nutritional interventions for vulnerable groups, including expansion of the ICDS program, nutrition and health education, programs for adolescent girls, better care of pregnant women, and control of micronutrient deficiencies. In addition, the policy calls for longer term institutional and structural changes through land reforms, increased and balanced food production, improved incomes, the PDS, education, information and communication, nutritional surveillance, and community participation. The policy also mentions the need to pay special attention to landless laborers, urban slum dwellers, hill people, seasonal nutritional problems, natural disasters, and the emerging problems of overnutrition among the affluent. It provides a framework for several nutrition-relevant sectors to work toward nutritional objectives and measure their achievements against nutritional goals. While implementation responsibility is spread across many sectors, the Department of Women and Child Development, which manages the ICDS program, is charged with monitoring progress toward achievement of the National Nutrition Goals.

A National Plan of Action for Nutrition (NPAN) specified actions for 14 concerned sectors (GOI, 1995).[16] The guiding principles of the NPAN include emphasis on the needy, sectoral coordination and convergence of services, participation of local governments and non-governmental organizations (NGOs), widespread information and education and social mobilization, detailed problem analysis, use of management information, and appropriate operational research. The NPAN discusses the mobilization of resources for nutrition interventions, placing responsibility with the state governments, local government bodies, and communities. A National Nutrition Council (NNC) was constituted in 1995 to oversee implementation of the NPAN, and state-level councils were also to be set up. While all these efforts are moving in the right direction, their potential has yet to be realized.

## Current Nutrition Programs: How Well Do They Work?

India will enter the 21st century with a supportive policy framework to tackle its immense malnutrition problem and several active programs that could succeed in reducing malnutrition significantly. The most important programs are the ICDS, the TPDS, food-for-work though JRY, NRY and EAS, the National Mid-day Meals Program (NMMP), and the micronutrient (iron-folate and vitamin A distribution and salt iodization) schemes. These programs aim to reach significant segments of India's undernourished population, such as poor households through the PDS and employment schemes, young children and mothers through the ICDS and health efforts, and school children through the NMMP. Brief reviews of each program are provided below. This report does not deal with the functioning, expenditures, or impact of wages provided through JRY, NRY, or EAS, nor with India's credit programs for the poor, the Integrated Rural Development Programme (IRDP), and the program for Development of Women and Children in Rural Areas (DWCRA). Although these programs may have nutritional impacts, these would derive from increased incomes and consumption expenditure.

There are few direct private sector efforts for nutritional improvement among the poor.[17] Some NGOs concerned with health have focused on the treatment or prevention of malnutrition among women and young children, and some broad-based development efforts have, for example, supported community nutrition measures, such as grain banks or food distribution. In the aggregate, however, these efforts reach a minuscule proportion of the country's poor, and would need to be multiplied several hundredfold to have a significant impact on India's malnutrition problem. In the short term, useful efforts would increase the attention of private medical practitioners to nutrition, focus the media on malnutrition and its effects, and disseminate information about successful NGO programs.

## Targeted Food Supplementation

*The Integrated Child Development Services Program (ICDS).* The ICDS program provides six services to 0–6-year-old children and mothers: supplementary feeding; immunization against preventable childhood diseases; health checkups and referral; health and nutrition education to adult women; and preschool education to 3–6-year-olds. Although the 0–6-year-old population of areas covered by the ICDS program is already 63 million, and the population of pregnant and lactating women is 13.6 million, only 30 million children and 5.2 million mothers are actually covered by supplementary feeding and 15 million 3–6-year-olds by preschool education. Coverage figures are not available for the other services. The ICDS also includes, in fewer than 10 percent of the 4,200 program blocks, schemes for adolescent girls' nutrition, health, awareness, and skill development; in some areas it has been linked with women's income-generating programs. All of the ICDS's services are delivered through a village center, the *anganwadi,* by a trained village woman who is assisted periodically in the health tasks by an Auxiliary Nurse Midwife (ANM) from the health subcenter.

The program is targeted to poor areas and, increasingly, to poor households. Program guidelines call for the food supplements, which are limited to 40 percent of the expected beneficiary population of an *anganwadi,* to be given preferentially to children and pregnant women from households at high risk of malnutrition—those of landless laborers, marginal farmers, scheduled castes, or tribes. The adolescent girls' and women's programs are intended to improve health and nutrition over the longer term through improvements in women's skills and access to resources. However, evaluations of the ICDS have found its impact on nutritional status to be limited (NFI, 1988; NIPCCD, 1992).[18, 19] The reasons for this include:

- Inadequate coverage of children below three years of age, those at greatest risk of malnutrition, and women and children living in hamlets

- Irregular food supply, irregular feeding, and inadequate rations

- Poor nutrition education of mothers (and none of families) to encourage improved feeding practices in the home and other relevant behavioral changes

- Inadequate training of workers, particularly in nutrition, growth monitoring, and communication

• *Anganwadi* worker (AWW) overload and weak and unsupportive supervision of AWWs, resulting in the neglect of crucial nutrition-related tasks

• Poor linkages between the ICDS program and the health system

In general the quality of the ICDS services is low. Although the services are much in demand, they are generally poorly delivered and uncoordinated. Worker training, in-service supervision, community support—indeed, community involvement in any sense—remain major gaps. With some exceptions, *anganwadi* facilities and environments are sorely inadequate, and the program does not inspire the good health, hygiene, and nutrition-related behaviors that are so essential to changing the status of children and women in poor households. To make a significant impact on nutrition and health, a great number of improvements are needed in the ICDS. Chapter 4 discusses these improvements.

*The National Mid-day Meals Programme (NMMP).* Initiated in 1995, the NMMP aims to increase primary school attendance and retention as well as improve the nutritional status and learning achievements of school children, generally in the 6–11-year-old age group. Some states—Andhra Pradesh, for example—emphasize the education of young girls through this program. The NMMP purportedly covers 91 million children, but the actual number fed is far fewer. School meals are provided in many areas in five states, while take-home rations are the norm in the majority of states. About 23 percent of the GOI education budget in 1997/98 and 16 percent in 1998/99 was earmarked for this program.[20] The program is currently short of funds, and continuation of its existing coverage is uncertain.

While the NMMP is believed to have increased the numbers of children attending school, its impact on nutritional status and cognitive development among the children is unknown. In other countries, school feeding has been found to increase learning achievement when provided as a breakfast to hungry children rather than as a noon meal. The NMMP strategy, which provides a child who has attended school regularly with a take-home ration of 3 kilograms of dry cereal, will have no impact whatsoever on the nutritional status of that child unless she or he consumes the food. To enhance nutrition and health status, food intake would need to be assured and accompanied by deworming, vitamin A and iron, and control of infections. These improvements in the NMMP would require state commitment to providing cooked meals at school, substantially increased management capacity, improvements in the school health program, and a larger quantity of resources than is currently available from either GOI or the state governments. Most countries have found universal school feeding programs unsustainable.

An objective evaluation of the NMMP is urgently required to measure its impact on enrollment, retention, and learning. This would provide the basis for necessary programmatic changes. But even without such an evaluation, given GOI and state resource constraints, there is a strong case for area targeting of the NMMP, for example, to districts chosen on the basis of low school attendance and high poverty ratios. In addition, in blocks not covered by the ICDS, program resources could be reallocated to younger children attending preschool centers run by the Department of Education, as they are usually more malnourished than primary school-aged children.

## Micronutrient Programs

*The National Nutritional Anemia Control Programme.* This program aims to reduce anemia among women of reproductive age and preschool children by providing iron-folate supplements, identifying and treating cases of severe anemia, and promoting the consumption of iron rich foods. In 1992, about 50 percent of Indian women received iron-folate supplements during prenatal care, although significant differences in coverage were found between urban and rural areas, age groups, educational status, and number of children per woman (IIPS, 1995).[21] The majority of poor women do not obtain adequate supplementation. Major shortages of iron-folate tablets have plagued the program continuously. Other problems include lack of worker motivation to distribute tablets and inadequate education of women and communities about their value—many women who receive the tablets do not consume them. As a result, India's very high rates of anemia persist, especially among pregnant women, and the impact of severe anemia on birth weight and maternal mortality is profound.

*The Vitamin A Prophylaxis Programme.* This program targets children between one and five years of age for a six-month dose of 200,000 International Units (IU) of vitamin A, and 6–11-month-old infants for a 100,000 IU dose. Therapeutic doses are given to those with detected deficiencies, and the program promotes improved dietary intake of foods rich in vitamin A. The Ministry of Health reported 68 percent coverage of 6–11-month-olds, and 25 percent coverage of 1—5-year-olds in 1996, but field reports suggest that actual coverage is considerably lower. Persistent shortages of vitamin A restrict the program, along with poor logistics and low community awareness. The ICDS has the potential to address at least the latter two problems.

*The National Iodine Deficiency Disorders Control Programme.* Having concentrated largely on ensuring the iodization of salt, this program is the most successful of the micronutrient programs. Yet production of iodized salt still falls woefully short of requirements, and quality control and trans-

portation remain bottlenecks. Although most states have banned the sale
of noniodized salt, it is still available widely, even in goiter-endemic areas.
The poor probably benefit least from this measure, as they are more likely
to consume unprocessed salt.

## Food Subsidy Programs

*The Public Distribution System (PDS).* India spends approximately 0.7 percent of GDP on food subsidies, including 0.5 percent on the PDS, which is
essentially untargeted (Radhakrishna, 1997).[22] Begun in the late 1950s to
support grain prices and assure buffer stocks when supplies fell short, the
PDS provides cereals and other essential items to card holders at subsidized rates. There are 400,000 Fair Price Shops throughout the country, up
from about 48,000 in 1960, supplied with centrally issued food grains
through the Food Corporation of India (FCI) and state procurement. The
program purportedly covers 85 percent of the people in the country, although the actual coverage is closer to 60 percent. The amount of foodgrain
distributed reached 20 million metric tons in 1997.

    While the PDS has been an important buffer against local food short-
ages, in many respects it has fallen short of providing food security to the
poor. It has been inadequately targeted, with a large number of beneficiaries actually coming from nonpoor households. Many of the poorer states
do not obtain the requisite quantities to cover their needy populations.
They take less than their share of supplies from the PDS mainly because of
a weak administrative capacity and the inability to move the food stocks.
There are serious leakages in the program, with supplies often finding
their way to the open market. The PDS is a high-cost operation relative to
the caloric support it provides: it costs about three times as much for the
PDS to provide a given number of calories to a household, compared with
the ICDS (Subbarao, 1990).[23] Most important, as late as 1997 the poor's
access to the PDS proved extremely limited, particularly in the most pov-
erty-stricken states (Radhakrishna and Subbarao, 1997).[24]

    *The Targeted Public Distribution System (TPDS).* In early 1997 the Central
Government introduced the Targeted PDS (TPDS) to ensure better coverage of households below the poverty line. Under the TPDS, BPL households are given a special identity card to obtain up to 10 kilograms of rice
or wheat per month at half the issue price. The Central Government will
allot adequate stocks to each state to cover the requirement for BPL households and, in most states, it will allocate additional amounts for those above
the poverty line as a transitory measure. The TPDS guidelines imply that
the second, nontargeted channel will be phased out gradually. While the
TPDS is designed to improve food supplies in the poorest households, it
has not gone far enough in a number of ways. The quantity of subsidized

grain provided amounts to a marginal supplement of 100 calories per person per day, much less than the estimated gap of poor people in rural areas. Secondly, in most states the PDS will still provide large quantities of subsidized food to nonpoor households, although this food could be targeted to needy children and mothers, for example, through the ICDS program. While politicians may waver at such reallocation, it is likely that more rural poor households will be helped immediately through the ICDS than through the TPDS because of its wider reach and targeted nature. Finally, it is unclear how the TPDS will plug leakages, particularly in the absence of a rigorous monitoring system.

India's foodgrain production has continued to increase fairly steadily, although population growth has eroded these gains somewhat. Per capita availability of food grains was 384 kilograms in 1960 and 464 kilograms in 1996. Unfortunately, the production of pulses, an important constituent of the vegetarian Indian diet, has fallen from 65.5 kilograms per capita to 34 kilograms in the same period, although availability has been boosted somewhat by imports. To ensure proper nutrition, adequate quantities of pulses or other protein-rich foods such as milk, eggs, or meat, which are also in short supply, must become more widely accessible, requiring increased production and improved distribution and consumption. Unless the prices of these commodities are reduced substantially—through vastly increased availability—they will remain out of the reach of the poor.

There is little independent corroboration of the extent to which the employment programs have supplemented the incomes and food available to the poor, although they are intended for this purpose. The programs are unfortunately fraught with leakages so that official data on the number of person-days of work cannot be assumed to accrue fully to the poor. The efforts of the employment programs to provide household food support by part payment in grain have been poorly implemented, and the programs have also fallen short of meeting other nutritionally relevant objectives, such as ensuring that 30 percent of beneficiaries are women, or raising participant families above the poverty line.

## What Is Wrong in the Aggregate?

Although we have pointed out the main deficiencies in each of the nutrition-related programs being implemented in India, it is also necessary to ask why the programs taken together have failed to combat malnutrition successfully. Each program appears well conceived, but in most cases implementation has been weak, particularly with regard to ensuring the access of the poor; and there are virtually no synergies between programs. Overall, the direct nutrition programs are insufficient to the task, uncoordinated, lack regular monitoring and evaluation, and show limited impact. If the current programs were targeted properly, rationalized, and improved in quality, they could succeed in substantially reducing malnutrition within the next two decades, particularly in the context of India's projected economic growth over this period. Recent developments in India, such as economic reforms, globalization processes, and the high skill-intensity of demand for labor, may increase the poor's vulnerability to shocks, and emphasize the need to strengthen programs such as the ICDS and the TPDS.

Although the nutrition-specific actions are embedded in a broader policy framework that emphasizes employment-intensive economic growth, greater access to social services, and specific poverty alleviation measures, the potential synergies among these wider efforts and the direct nutrition programs remain largely undeveloped. The Department of Women and Child Development has not been able to coordinate the many institutions involved in the nutrition-related sectors. Indeed, without adequate support from the National Nutrition Council, such coordination is unlikely. Furthermore, unless the department itself is strengthened, it cannot play a more forceful role in advocating enhanced efforts for nutrition.

The grinding poverty of rural (and urban slum) India suggests that BPL households need to be reached by *all* of the programs mentioned above: the employment schemes and the TPDS to ensure adequate income and food availability to poor households; ICDS to care for the nutrition and health care needs of vulnerable women and children; and the NMMP to provide school children with both the incentive and nutritional support to learn. However, the affordability of all these programs is questionable and, therefore, in the context of inadequate resources, it is necessary in the next section of this report to examine their relative costs and contributions to achieving nutritional objectives.

## Government Spending on Nutrition Programs

*Nutrition Spending by the States.* Table 1 provides information on nutrition spending in 12 major states during 1992–95 as a percentage of their state domestic product (SDP). Nutrition spending varies widely by state, with no apparent correlation with the level of need, as measured by either the extent of poverty, the prevalence of malnutrition, or the SDP.[25] Of the 12 major states for which data are available, 9 spent less than 0.25 percent of SDP, Orissa and Gujarat spent between 0.25 percent and 0.5 percent, and only Tamil Nadu spent more than 0.5 percent of SDP.

Examining nutrition expenditure per child reveals a similar picture. Among the 12 states surveyed, per child expenditure in 1994/95 ranged from a high of Rupees (Rs.) 317 in Tamil Nadu to Rs. 31 in Rajasthan and West Bengal. Expenditures per malnourished child in the 12 states ranged from Rs. 732 in Tamil Nadu to Rs. 36 in West Bengal. Radhakrishna and Narayana (1993)[26] reported that per child expenditure on nutrition was also very low in the poor states of Uttar Pradesh and Bihar throughout the period 1974–90. Tamil Nadu accounted for 7 percent of the malnourished children in the 12 states in Table 1, but for 37 per cent of the total nutrition expenditure. On the other hand, Rajasthan, Madhya Pradesh, and West Bengal accounted for half of the malnourished children in the 12 states but spent only about one-fourth of the total expenditure in 1994–95. In summary, most of the 12 states were not allocating resources to nutrition commensurate with their malnutrition or poverty problem.

Public spending on nutrition programs is a necessary but insufficient measure for reducing malnutrition, which is a function of many variables. For example, Rajasthan has less malnutrition than Tamil Nadu despite spending much less as a proportion of SDP (see Table 1). Similarly, there is little correlation between state-level spending on health programs and levels of mortality. Nutritional status, like health status, is determined by multiple factors: income and poverty, educational attainment, gender equity, and historical rates of investment in the social sectors and antipoverty programs, to name only a few.

*Total Government Spending on Nutrition.* The GOI and state spending on direct nutrition programs consists predominantly of the ICDS, the NMMP, and micronutrient programs. Figure 1 provides a rough estimate of the average expenditures on these programs for the period 1995 to 1998. India spends a considerably larger amount on indirect nutrition programs, even if only the cereal subsidy component of the PDS and the foodgrain component of the centrally funded employment programs are included (Figure 1).

India spends considerably less on nutritional programs than is needed to reduce malnutrition among children under five years of age and pregnant and lactating women. From 1985 to 1990, the average annual expenditure by the states and the GOI on direct nutrition programs (mainly the ICDS and the NMMP) amounted to 0.15 percent of GNP (World Bank, 1993).[27] Spending has increased in the 1990s due to the expansion of the ICDS and the NMMP in 1995 and now amounts to approximately 0.19 percent of GNP. In contrast, Sri Lanka, a country with a reputation for considerable success in reducing the level of malnutrition, spent about 1 percent of its GNP on direct nutrition programs during the mid-1980s. Given the magnitude of its malnutrition crisis, India should anticipate spending a minimum of 0.5 percent of GNP on direct nutrition programs, or more than double its current spending.

Although we have not considered the importance of economic growth and employment, agriculture, women's programs, education, health, water and sanitation to improved nutrition, India is not spending enough on

**Table 1. Nutrition Spending in Selected States, 1992–95**

| State | Population below poverty line (percent) 1993–94 | Severely and moderately malnourished children (percent) 1992–93 | Net annual state domestic product (Rs. per capita) 1994–95 | Nutrition spending as a percentage of state domestic product | | |
|---|---|---|---|---|---|---|
| | | | | 1992–93 | 1993–94 | 1994–95 |
| Andhra Pradesh | 23 | 49 | 5718 | 0.11 | 0.10 | 0.11 |
| Assam | 41 | 50 | 4973 | 0.11 | 0.12 | 0.17 |
| Gujarat | 24 | 50 | 8164 | 0.31 | 0.31 | 0.29 |
| Haryana | 25 | 38 | 9037 | 0.17 | 0.17 | 0.16 |
| Karnataka | 33 | 54 | 6315 | 0.08 | 0.08 | 0.10 |
| Kerala | 25 | 29 | 5768 | 0.10 | 0.09 | 0.12 |
| Madhya Pradesh | 43 | 57 | 4544 | 0.20 | 0.16 | 0.18 |
| Maharashtra | 37 | 54 | 9806 | 0.08 | 0.08 | 0.08 |
| Orissa | 49 | 53 | 4114 | 0.32 | 0.33 | 0.36 |
| Rajasthan | 27 | 42 | 5257 | 0.09 | 0.12 | 0.13 |
| Tamil Nadu | 35 | 48 | 6670 | 0.62 | 0.53 | 0.58 |
| West Bengal | 36 | 57 | 5541 | 0.07 | 0.08 | 0.08 |

*Note:* Nutrition spending figures include GOI and state government expenditures on the ICDS, the NMMP, and other nutrition programs.
*Sources:* State government budgets; Planning Commission, "Expert Group on Estimation of Proportion and Number of Poor, 1993–94"; and International Institute for Population Sciences. 1995. *National Family Health Survey (MCH and Family Planning), India, 1992–93.* Bombay: Government of India. 1996. National Sample Survey Organization. *Nutritional Intake in India, Fifth Quinquennial Survey on Consumer Expenditure.*[28] Department of Statistics.

## Figure 1. Average Annual Total Government Spending on Direct and Indirect Nutrition Programs, 1995–98

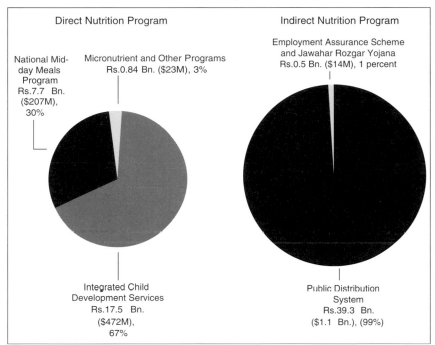

*Note:* The ICDS costs include the GOI and state-financed supplementary food expenditures; the NNMP costs are all GOI expenditures; micronutrient and other program costs include GOI expenditures on National Iodine Deficiency Disorders Control Program plus 5 percent of the Department of Family Welfare budget to cover the iron and vitamin A distribution programs; the PDS costs are the total cereal subsidy, and EAS/JRY costs are for the food grains provided.

*Sources:* Central Government expenditure budgets, departmental budgets, and Economic Survey, 1997–98. Government of India. 1998a. *Economic Survey 1997–98*. New Delhi: Ministry of Finance, Economic Division.[29]

direct nutrition programs by any standard. What about the composition of spending and the quality and impact of each program? Is India allocating resources appropriately among programs? What are the returns on these investments? And, given scarce resources, how might these returns be increased? There is clearly a need to increase the size of the nutrition resource pie; but there is also scope to improve the returns on investments, and to reallocate resources to enhance effectiveness. The ICDS has the greatest potential for bringing about the behavioral changes in the health, caring, and feeding practices required to reduce malnutrition among women and small children. Similarly, the TPDS, if it reached the poor, could have a major impact on household food security, a significant part of the malnutrition problem. Chapter 4 addresses the quality and impact of the programs and suggests options for change that could increase the returns on program investments from a nutritional perspective. It then suggests how the pie might be better divided to deal with the malnutrition crisis.

# Chapter 4

# Meeting the Crisis:
# What India Must Do

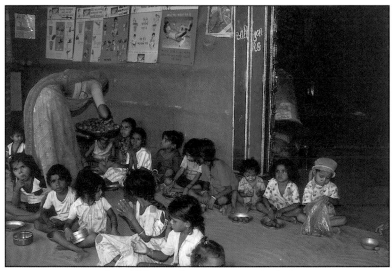

*Feeding children in the ICDS program in Gujarat*

India's nutrition policies and plans have been generally sound, but their implementation has been woefully inadequate. Two essential ingredients for success are missing: adequate and sustained commitment to the actions required to deal with the malnutrition problem, and the capacity to implement, evaluate, and revise the programs aimed at reducing malnutrition. Meeting the National Nutrition Goals set for the year 2000 even by 2010 demands action and demonstrated success in four principal areas. First, the country must develop the leadership structure and administrative capacity to ensure commitment to and management of the programs required to deal with the massive challenge. This encompasses the policy, planning, and implementation structure and the institutional and individual capacities necessary to make it work effectively. Second, the ICDS program must greatly improve the quality of its services and their impact on vulnerable groups. Both the quality of services and their impact must be regularly monitored and evaluated, and improvements must be made continuously. Third, the health sector must give higher

29

priority to malnutrition and ensure that its actions have far greater impact on the problem than at present. And fourth, India must do better at providing food security to the poor at the community and household level. Sustained success in these four areas is essential if India is to deal effectively with the crisis of malnutrition and prevent both its human and financial resources from wasting away. This chapter discusses why these actions are critical and how they can be achieved. It ends by estimating the resource needs for each strategy, and for the set of actions as a whole.

## Building Commitment and Capacity

*Political Commitment Is Crucial.* India needs to manifest greater political will to combat its malnutrition problem. Although a National Nutrition Council was constituted in 1995, it has yet to convene, and the proposed state nutrition councils have yet to be established. Such a policy structure is vital and must actively lead, monitor, and sustain national, state, and local action to address malnutrition across the many sectors involved. And it must be ably assisted by expanded and strengthened Departments of Women and Child Development (DWCD), especially at the central government level. A high level of commitment and technical and managerial expertise at central and state levels are required to rebuild India's once substantial capacity for nutrition training, research, and evaluation. This will require renewed attention to institutions, such as the National Institute of Nutrition, and the provision of incentives to attract the best and brightest Indians to careers in nutrition. India needs to mount a massive and sustained effort to inform policy-makers, the public, the professions, the media, and citizens from all walks of life that the country's future social and economic development vitally depends on reducing the scourge of malnutrition. Above all, it will require the strong determination of policy-makers, program managers, functionaries, and beneficiaries to increase the quality, cost-effectiveness, and impact of nutrition programs. Some states, such as Tamil Nadu, and agencies, such as CARE, boast impressive records of actively dealing with malnutrition, providing models for strengthening the policy, planning, and implementation framework for improved nutrition services.

*Strong Nutrition Institutions Are Critical.* India's institutional capacity in nutrition began to decline in the 1980s, and today it is deplorably weak. Earlier, India had a vibrant and internationally renowned set of nutrition institutions. Nutrition activities were well developed in agricultural universities, colleges of home science, medical colleges, and national institutes such as the All-India Institute of Public Health and Hygiene in

Calcutta. The National Institute of Nutrition (NIN) was at the forefront of international research and training in nutrition science.

India needs to recognize openly the current gap and provide the resources to build institutions capable of dealing with its vast and varied malnutrition problems. The ultimate goal must be to ensure that there is sufficient capacity to undertake the policy-making, program design, implementation, training, monitoring, and research tasks required to address malnutrition in the country. There is a pressing need to document the nutritional situation, study its determinants and consequences, design appropriate interventions, and manage their implementation within the context of 21st century science and political economy. There is also an urgent need to train people, from village-level workers to medical specialists and policy-makers, and to greatly expand public awareness of malnutrition through communications and education. Institutions are needed in every major state of the country, as identification of nutritional problems and program responses must be region-specific. Rebuilding capacity should begin by mapping existing institutions and their capabilities and measuring these against what is needed to revitalize nutrition efforts. To understand both the quantitative dimensions and qualitative nature of the rebuilding required, it will be necessary to carry out needs assessments of key institutions and an overall human resource planning exercise. Beyond this, a phased approach should be adopted to increase the size and number of institutions and to bring about qualitative improvements in existing ones.

*Leadership and Networking.* Among nutrition institutions, NIN and the National Institute of Public Cooperation and Child Development (NIPCCD) could be instrumental in expanding capacity in both research and training. They should be granted autonomous status and financed separately from the Indian Council of Medical Research and the DWCD, respectively, where, in recent years, they have not received the support required. They could then catalyze a network of institutions concerned with nutrition. These institutions must be action-oriented. There is vast scope in India for new programs at the local level to deal with malnutrition, and for improved management of existing programs. Similarly, the Food and Nutrition Bureau, which was earlier under the Department of Food but has now been brought under the DWCD, must be revitalized to play a greater role, particularly in ensuring appropriate food production and availability for nutritional improvement. Sustained effort to develop nutrition leadership among all these institutions and competitive processes to allocate resources to innovative and effective initiatives are required. Upgraded equipment and methods of teaching are necessary to encourage a new—and modern—generation of nutrition scientists, practitioners, and policy analysts.

There is also a need to change the gender stereotype of the nutrition professional and attract more men to the field while at the same time ensuring that women are well represented in leadership positions.

*Building Capacity for Nutrition.* The ICDS requires that large numbers of *anganwadi* workers, supervisors, and officers be trained initially, and provided with refresher training and short courses in special skills and topics. The NIPCCD has carried out assessments of the training capacity for the ICDS in different states. Completion of these assessments and an overall mapping, along with rigorous analyses of the number of persons requiring training, will determine how many more training centers need to be established for the different cadres, and where these should be located. The DWCD aims to decentralize responsibility for training and its planning, which is a welcome move. In addition, improvements need to be made urgently and continuously in the content and quality of training and monitored for effectiveness and impact. The establishment of a streamlined management information system for training in the ICDS is long overdue. The national training component of the 1999 World Bank-assisted Woman and Child Development Project provides both a ready framework and finances for these tasks.

Basic health workers and auxiliary nurse midwives also require solid training in nutrition. This calls for the development of nutrition curricula to be incorporated into their current training and requires a similar assessment of training capacity, quality, and the useful outcomes of this training. In particular, the joint training of the ICDS and health workers requires additional capacity, development of innovative methods and materials, and extensive follow-up.

Strengthening medical education to address malnutrition is critical to the development of adequate nutrition services in the health system as well as to the revitalization of nutrition research in the field, medical colleges, and hospitals. Curriculum development, new training methodologies, and grant/award programs for practical applications are required. Doctors must be trained in nutrition, and their involvement in nutrition diagnosis, education, and monitoring must be fostered. Doctors and other workers must at least be able to manage moderate and severe malnutrition, counsel parents of sick children on proper feeding and care, and ensure that all pregnant women receive iron-folate supplements. Medical colleges need to play a far greater role in community nutrition beyond their current role of training and research for the ICDS. Nutrition must become part of the agenda of the health sector at every level.

*Research for Action.* Currently there is a paucity of nutrition research, whether policy, field, or laboratory, although there are many institutions in the country with interests in nutrition. Increasing the budgets of these institutions is required to reinvigorate research, particularly practical, action-oriented research. It is essential that institutions assume a greater role in programs such as the ICDS and conduct relevant operational research and policy studies. A program of grants is also needed for demographic and social science research institutes, non-governmental organizations (NGOs), and other field-based organizations to develop nutrition interests and capabilities.

Priority areas for research include:

• Program-driven nutrition studies, i.e., operational research that emanates directly from constraints to program effectiveness, for example, in reducing low birth weight and anemia

• Analysis of nutritional needs at the local level and means by which programs (TPDS, ICDS, health, water and sanitation, etc.) can be designed to meet these needs

• Nutrition status measurement and determinants analyses, including surveys and qualitative studies

• Scientific and technological research, especially on major problems such as anemia and nutrition-infection relationships

• Studies on the nutrition consequences of new economic, including agriculture, and social policies and programs

• Economic studies, such as cost-benefit and cost-effectiveness analyses, of nutrition interventions.

*Nutrition Monitoring.* India needs to establish a broad-based, efficient system to collect and analyze nutrition data for use in decision-making and advocacy. The emphasis must be on collecting relevant and manageable amounts of high-quality information, not on large quantities liable to remain unused. Nutrition status data must be collected and made available at regular intervals, at least annually. The National Nutrition Monitoring Bureau (NNMB) was an excellent idea in this regard, but it has not been as active and rigorous as desirable. A carefully targeted and reliable system is urgently needed, using the best data collection, computerization, and analysis methods. This should be linked to the National Sample Survey (with appropriate modifications of this effort) and to the ICDS program. The ICDS method for gathering data on children and mothers, and reporting these monthly, urgently needs to be improved. Although the concurrent evaluation of the ICDS recently piloted by the National Council of Applied Economic Research (NCAER) may be useful, it is no substitute for a well-functioning monitoring system (NCAER, 1998).[30] An expert task force has been constituted to develop a Nutrition Surveillance System for the country, and the Food and Nutrition Bureau is developing district nutrition profiles using several relevant indicators, but neither of these efforts would be necessary if the NNMB and the ICDS systems were strengthened and expanded. A high-level authority, such as the National Nutrition Council, should receive and review nutrition data at least annually and ensure progress in reducing malnutrition. Appropriate nutrition data should be used for policy-making, program planning, local interventions, and focused research.

*Advocacy and Communication.* There is currently little effort in the country to advocate better nutrition or communicate nutrition messages of vital importance to the public. Extension workers in agriculture (in addition to health and the ICDS), schools, and mass media, including national and regional broadcast media, are some of the channels that could be used to promote awareness of nutrition as a community and national development challenge. Programs that educate individuals and families about good nutrition and the consequences of malnutrition, as well as efforts to inform policy-makers, planners, and managers, are sorely needed. A structured program of advocacy meetings is required for government officials and leaders at the national, state, and district levels to ensure a common frame of reference for understanding malnutrition and how to deal with it.

*Institute an Annual Progress Review.* Until the malnutrition crisis is overcome, India needs to conduct an annual review of progress against its quantified National Nutrition Goals. This would be best accomplished by holding a high-visibility national workshop annually, attended by the country's top policy-makers and leaders. Such a rigorous assessment could be carried out each year during National Nutrition Week, with heavy media coverage. The GOI should also consider instituting an annual National Nutrition Award for the state or district that is most innovative and successful in reducing malnutrition.

## Enhancing the Quality and Impact of the ICDS Program

The ICDS covers approximately 70 percent of the country's development blocks. It is relatively well targeted to the poorest areas, especially those populated by India's most downtrodden groups: the scheduled castes and tribes (Chatterjee, 1997).[31] The ICDS program's most important assets include a holistic approach to child development and the use of locally recruited, village-level workers. Beneficiaries value the program's preschool and child-feeding features.

Unfortunately, the ICDS is not having the intended nutritional impact on young children and mothers nationwide. This is principally because its effective national coverage is low. For example, the ICDS provides supplementary feeding for only 30 million of the country's approximately 162 million 0–6-year-olds, or less than one child in five. If the feeding were well targeted to the poor, estimated to be one-third of the population, it would still reach less than half of those in need. Even within the covered blocks, less than 50 percent of children are reached, and these may not include the most needy. For many reasons the program's main focus gradually has become food supplementation and preschool education for 3–6-year-olds, to the neglect of children under 3, especially those aged 6–24 months. Moreover, as the 1992 NIPCCD evaluation demonstrated, ICDS had not brought about the behavioral changes necessary among families to prevent malnutrition in young children or low birthweight babies. It is important to note that no monitoring and evaluation system exists that can reliably gauge the impact of the ICDS on its primary objectives.

The ICDS is a highly centralized program, and its top-down approach constitutes a major reason why the program's intended community ownership and management are virtually nonexistent (Chatterjee, 1996).[32] The program is seen by beneficiaries, bureaucrats, and politicians alike as a government program providing feeding and preschool education. In addition, the ICDS program has followed a standard approach to implementation in each development block, although substantial variations in malnutrition, and its social and economic determinants, call for flexibility and responses tailored to local needs, cultural preferences, and capabilities. In 1997 the GOI began to devolve centrally sponsored schemes to the states. The ICDS was not included in the first wave of devolution, but the DWCD has begun decentralizing its activities, starting with the key area of worker training.

The GOI has endeavored to implement the key recommendations of the NIPCCD evaluation, but efforts to improve the quality of the ICDS have thus far been overshadowed by the priority given to universalizing program coverage. The ICDS needs to improve its quality, effectiveness, efficiency, and impact, ensuring its sustainability for as long as necessary. How can the ICDS be strengthened for the 21st century to make a major impact on malnutrition in the next decade? Reaching young children at risk, and the women most likely to have low birthweight babies, is the key to increasing the impact and cost-effectiveness of the ICDS and thus its contribution, as India's major direct nutrition program, to reducing malnutrition. Given the extent of the problems revealed in the NIPCCD evaluation and numerous other studies, the case for reform is strong. The changes need to achieve at least the following four objectives:

• Improved targeting, especially to reach those children under two and pregnant women who are most at risk of malnutrition

• Greatly enhanced quality of services and impact, particularly on behavioral change

•  A reliable monitoring and evaluation system as soon as possible

• Community ownership and management of the program

Until these improvements are achieved, the ICDS program should not be expanded beyond the current number of blocks. The area targeting approach has ensured that the neediest blocks are covered. Available resources should be used instead to improve the coverage of villages and hamlets within these blocks, and the quality of services. Rigorous criteria such as coverage with growth monitoring, deliveries by trained attendants, improved nutritional status, and birthweight monitoring should be used to determine whether program quality has improved sufficiently.

*Reaching Those Most at Risk.* There is now a consensus within India and globally that reaching children aged 6–24 months and pregnant women most at risk is critical to preventing malnutrition. These groups need a few specific health interventions, nutrition support, and appropriate information. No major program in the world has succeeded in meeting the health and nutrition needs of these target groups and simultaneously succeeded in imparting preschool education to 3–6-year-olds through a single worker. The ICDS has also failed to do so. The TINP reduced severe and, to some extent, moderate malnutrition by devoting a worker to only 6–36-month-old children and pregnant and lactating women.[33] When preschool education was added to the program in a second phase, a separate worker was employed. The single overburdened *anganwadi* worker (AWW) of the ICDS cannot simultaneously manage preschool education and supplementary feeding at the *anganwadi* center and also undertake the outreach necessary to provide care to 6–24-month-old children and pregnant women at risk.[34]

The GOI–Bank workshop held in June 1998 produced several proposed options for refocusing the ICDS on the young child and pregnant woman, including the following:

• A second worker for preschool education, selected and financed by the village *panchayat*

• A village-level health worker, financed by the community or the health system

• The training of adolescent girls, women, youth, *dais*, teachers, and others to assist the AWW

No solution is likely to be applicable to all situations, but it is imperative to adopt one of the above options or make some other change in order to achieve the ICDS's objectives of preventing malnutrition in young children and reducing the number of low birthweight babies. Where village *panchayats* are strong, the second worker is likely to be the best option. Given the disappointing previous experience in India with the Community Health Worker program, the second option would be viable only where the health system can properly train and support such workers. The third option, with responsibility and accountability resting on no single individual, requires a high level of community cohesion and collaboration and would, therefore, only work in select locations.

A radical alternative is more likely to solve the problem of the AWW overload: separate services to 3–6-year-old children from those for 6–36-month-olds and pregnant and lactating women. The demand for preschool education, and for feeding 3–6-year-old children, could be met by a second worker in the ICDS or by devolving these services to the Department of Education or to local authorities. The District Primary Education Program (DPEP) already delivers preschool education services in some districts, and the feeding of 3–6-year-olds could become part of the National Mid-day Meals Program, as discussed below.

*Targeting and Sustainability*. The ICDS program's food costs now account for about two-thirds of the total cost of the program (Radhakrishna and others, 1998).[35] Virtually all states, with the exception of Tamil Nadu, consistently underfinance the food component, which is solely their responsibility, because of its high cost and logistical difficulties. This results in frequent food shortages. The NIPCCD evaluation reported that disruptions in food distribution occurred for periods of over 90 days in 27 percent of *anganwadis*, and that the average duration without food was 64 days per *anganwadi* per year (out of an intended total of 300 feeding days). Evaluations also show that many of the children and women most in need are not reached.[36] With progress towards universalization of the ICDS, many states are finding the burden of providing food according to the ICDS norms increasingly difficult to bear. On the other hand, it is politically difficult for states *not* to provide food to children under six, when the NMMP is attempting to feed all public primary school children in the country.

Convergence of the ICDS and the NMMP programs offers an attractive policy option from the standpoint of both preschool education and nutrition. Given the chronic underfunding of NMMP, a means of targeting the program will have to be found, as suggested earlier in Chapter 3. In addition to area targeting of the NMMP to enhance its cost-effectiveness and impact on its primary educational goals, targeting the feeding on younger children will enhance its impact on nutrition and, through that, on learning. In fact, scientific evidence suggests that feeding very young children and preschoolers, rather than 6–11-year-olds, will have a greater impact on child learning and overall development. Targeting food distribution to the most needy and most likely to benefit, both in the ICDS (the 0–3-year-olds) and the NMMP (the 3–6-year-olds), and ensuring that lean periods are covered on a priority basis, will also contribute to solving the problem of the mounting costs of these feeding programs, which are unlikely to be sustained even at current levels.

*Enhancing the Quality and Impact of the ICDS.* The principal reason that the ICDS is not covering children under-two and pregnant women is that the AWW cannot reach these target groups through home visits principally— while she is burdened with child-feeding, preschool education, record-keeping, and many other duties at the *anganwadi.* Nor can she focus on communicating key messages to mothers to effect behavior changes related to child care, breast-feeding, complementary feeding, prenatal care, anemia, etc. Once freed from the responsibility of supplementary feeding and preschool education, she will have time to care for those most at risk of malnutrition. But she will only be effective in bringing about behavioral change if she is better trained and supported for that role. The DWCD and the states are engaged in a major effort to enhance the training of the AWWs and other workers with support from the nationwide training component of the Woman and Child Development Project, approved by the Bank in June 1998. This represents a positive development. Strengthening the supportive supervision of the AWW is another indispensable requirement to increase the effectiveness of the ICDS in preventing malnutrition. If these objectives were achieved, the ICDS could reduce child malnutrition to the same level as the TINP, which lowered severe malnutrition rates by one-half in less than five years, and the ICDS could expect to reduce moderate malnutrition substantially.

*Decentralized Management and Community Ownership.* Once the ICDS has adopted strategies to ensure the coverage of very young children and pregnant women and the appropriate targeting of feeding, the next major step is to ensure a community context in which the strategies will flourish. To achieve community ownership, the ICDS must first devolve responsibility to the states in order to adapt the basic model to their particular problems and needs and take full charge of program management. In addition to the GOI's intention to devolve centrally sponsored schemes to the states and the ICDS's efforts to decentralize training, the emerging *panchayati raj* institutions, whose capability is growing with their responsibility for the social sectors, will make decentralization to communities more feasible now than ever before.

Below the state level, decentralized management could be achieved by many routes: delegating the implementation of the ICDS to the private sector or NGOs; setting up autonomous societies at the district or block levels; or devolving responsibility to the district, block and village *panchayats.* Neither the private sector nor NGOs offer a viable option because of the massive scale of services demanded by the size of the malnutrition problem. Private efforts can, however, complement the ICDS in important ways, notably by experimentation and dissemination of information about effective innovations.

Devolving implementation responsibility to district-level societies offers some promise. There are successful precedents for this in education (DPEP) and health ( blindness, leprosy, and tuberculosis programs). The district, averaging about 10 blocks nationwide, provides a sound organizational unit for the ICDS services, offering both a critical mass for cost-effective training programs and a reasonable span of managerial control. Organizing the ICDS services at the district level would offer a key advantage that organization at the state level would neglect, namely, an ability to adapt closely to local conditions.

The district approach might have five key features. First, it could formally involve the *Zilla Parishad* for the purpose of initiating community ownership. Second, it could operate through a registered society at the district level to provide administrative flexibility and accountability. Third, funding could pass to the registered society on a nationally equitable and transparent basis. Fourth, progress toward agreed upon and verified performance goals could provide the basis for continued funding. And fifth, considerable implementation flexibility could be encouraged to ensure that the ICDS better serves the needs of individual communities, thereby achieving program goals. An unerring focus on providing program benefits to the poor in all communities is essential.

## Strengthening Nutrition Action by the Health Sector

Improving nutrition in India now depends more than ever on effective action by the health sector. Indeed, this is imperative because further reductions in infant and child mortality will be difficult to achieve in the face of rampant malnutrition. The task is feasible because the basic skills and tools to break the nutrition-infection cycle, which critically determines malnutrition, are available to health workers. Moreover, improvements in water, sanitation, and personal hygiene depend on the health sector. Despite the recent improvements cited by Harsh Pal Singh Sachdev (1997),[37] the prevalence of low birth weight, usually estimated at one-third of births, is a huge barrier to further improvements in the nutrition and health status of children. Mothers must enter pregnancy in good nutritional status if they are to emerge from the birth process healthy and give birth to healthy infants. This, in turn, means that adolescent girls must receive care to ensure that they enter the reproductive period in good physical condition. These life-cycle goals are not currently being achieved in India, but they are achievable if a major effort is made by both families and programs. For example, in Gambia, a low-income African country, research demonstrated that low birth weight could be reduced by 50 percent and infant mortality by 40 percent through substantially increased food intake during the latter half of pregnancy (Ceesay and others, 1997).[38]

Collaboration between the ICDS and the health delivery system has improved in recent years. Most progress has been achieved in immunization, which has demonstrated successful collaboration between the AWW and the auxiliary nurse midwife (ANM). Despite its promise, this partnership has been less successful in identifying pregnancies early, detecting women at particular risk, providing prenatal care, and conveying vital health and nutritional messages to women. Far too many women at high risk escape the attention of the AWW and the ANM until late in pregnancy, or altogether. This reduces these women's chances of gaining sufficient weight, receiving supplementary food from the ICDS, and getting tetanus immunization and iron supplements, lowering the probability of good outcomes to their pregnancies. Improving the alliance between the village-based AWW, with a catchment population of around 1,000, and the ANM, with a population of approximately 7,000–8,000, will prove crucial to improving the role of the health sector in nutrition.

*Training in Nutrition.* Inadequate nutrition training of health personnel compounds the difficulty of ensuring effective nutrition-health collaboration. In India, as elsewhere, nutrition is a neglected topic in medical and nursing schools and among other health personnel. Progress in this area demands an integrated approach to nutrition and health. In the short term, the key priority is to strengthen the ANM training in nutrition. The ICDS has recently taken steps to strengthen and decentralize its training program, which should make the future AWW a more able partner to the ANM. But the ANM, who starts out with higher educational qualifications and is trained for a considerably longer period than the AWW, must receive complementary training to fulfill her nutrition-related role. In addition, these workers need joint protocols, joint training, and much better on-the-job supportive supervision.

Although malnutrition is associated with one-half of all child deaths, rural doctors are poorly equipped to deal with malnutrition. Individual doctors and the staff of primary health centers and community health centers must be able to quickly recognize nutritional disorders, manage low birth weight and malnutrition, and, above all, provide mothers and families the advice and assistance on breast-feeding, weaning, and caring practices that will prevent malnutrition.

*Reaching 6–24 Month-Olds and Pregnant Women.* The AWW must reach out to these two vulnerable groups. She must identify and bring to the care of the ANM those women and children who are most at risk of malnutrition and illness. The TINP came close to achieving this objective by emphasizing home visits and ensuring strong community involvement in the program. In addition to prenatal care, iron supplementation, and immunization, which are relatively easy services to deliver, the AWW and the ANM must provide adequate information and motivation to mothers to effect behavioral change.

*Reaching Adolescent Girls.* Ensuring that adolescent girls reach reproductive age with the best education and health and nutritional status possible is arguably the biggest challenge facing India's social sectors. Feasible approaches are yet to be discovered, and the initial efforts of the ICDS to reach adolescent girls have had mixed success. The ICDS is now attempting to reach this target group with iron supplements and periodic deworming, an effort deserving careful evaluation and appropriate strengthening. Indeed, this area demands good operational research, so that different approaches can be carefully assessed to determine which work best in different parts of the country. Of critical importance is the need to impart nutrition and health education to adolescent girls through the ICDS and health services.

*Decentralization.* Devolving responsibility to local communities for reaching all these groups is likely to achieve better results than those to date. This applies equally to the ICDS and Health and Family Welfare programs. The more communities become involved in the management of these problems, which have strong social underpinnings, the greater the likelihood of success, as demonstrated by some of the NGO programs and innovative public sector efforts. If the AWWs and the ANMs are accountable to local communities by, for example, having their stipends and salaries paid through the local *panchayat*, they are likely to be much more effective in reducing malnutrition in India.

What have been the main impediments to departments of Health and Family Welfare taking greater responsibility for nutrition? The current organizational arrangements create unnecessary barriers. While the Department of Women and Child Development, within the Ministry of Human Resource Development, is the central department for nutrition, with responsibility for the ICDS, the Ministry of Health and Family Welfare (MOHFW) commands key resources for interventions against malnutrition, including micronutrient fortification and supplementation programs. Furthermore, the MOHFW is divided into two departments, with the Department of Family Welfare responsible for Maternal and Child Health, including iron and vitamin A programs, and the Department of Health overseeing iodine deficiency disorders.

The organizational arrangements also differ by state, with some having combined and some separate components of Health and Family Welfare departments. In most states, as at the central government level, the ICDS and Health and Family Welfare departments are separate. In Gujarat and Sikkim, the ICDS combines with Health and Family Welfare, but coordination between these subdepartments is lacking. Given this division of responsibility at central and state levels, it is not surprising that collaboration suffers. The immediate need is for the Health and Family Welfare authorities to give far greater priority to nutrition. If this is not done, they are unlikely to achieve their health goals. Senior officers in charge of nutrition are needed in the departments of health, family welfare, and medical education. Once that commitment is evident, serious consideration should be given to merging the Reproductive and Child Health and the ICDS programs, which need to work seamlessly at the village level if either is to succeed in its mandate.

## Nutrition Security at the Community and Household Levels

For the vast majority of India's poor—more than 350 million people—malnutrition results from inadequate purchasing power. Despite five decades of poverty alleviation programs providing wage employment, subsidized credit, and food for work, the poor cannot look forward to the basic two square meals a day. While the malnutrition of young children and pregnant women, who are among the worst sufferers, can sometimes be alleviated by marginal reallocations of food within their households, it is imperative to improve the overall food security of poor households.

The TPDS offers great potential for providing extra food to poor households. Its success in reaching the poor needs to be carefully monitored—and accelerated. Anecdotal evidence suggests coverage of the poor is increasing in Uttar Pradesh and Bihar, but documentation of overall trends is lacking and urgently needed. The plan to issue new cards for households below the poverty line is important, and the program must not be swayed from this intention by political compulsions at any level. BPL households must be selected properly and transparently. In the past, other schemes with the express intention of targeting the poor (such as Andhra Pradesh's two-rupee rice scheme) were diluted by improper allocation of cards. There is ample evidence that when the nonpoor gain access to programs such as the PDS, the poor are pushed out. The failure of the Revamped TPDS is an indication that, despite good intentions, it remains difficult to get food supplies into poor areas.

There is another compelling reason to ensure appropriate targeting of cards and supplies. For the TPDS to have any nutritional impact, allocations to poor households must be increased. As described in Chapter 3, the current TPDS provision of 10 kilograms per household provides an additional 100 calories per person per day, which is inadequate for the poorest households. If the TPDS is to bring caloric levels for the poorest 30 percent from the current average of about 1,500 calories per person per day to even a modest average of 1,900 calories, a reasonable objective for the program, allocation of an additional 30 kilograms beyond the currently proposed amount per household is necessary. These allocations are based upon the assumption that these very poor households are likely to maximize their expenditure on food when it is highly subsidized. Providing additional grain allocations during the months when they are most needed by rural households, the preharvest and rainy seasons, constitutes an especially critical measure to prevent vulnerable children and pregnant women from declining in nutritional status and succumbing to disease and death during these periods.

However, there is grave danger that the TPDS, like its parent, the PDS, will be usurped in time by those who do not need to receive subsidized food. To prevent this, the government needs to design other safety mechanisms. For example, it could allocate the contracts for Fair Price Shops to community groups and cooperatives on a larger scale. Implementation of this strategy has witnessed some success in reaching the poor in some states, such as Andhra Pradesh, and Tamil Nadu in the south and Madhya Pradesh and Rajasthan in the north. In particular, women's groups have proved adept at managing the ration shops and ensuring more equitable access to the subsidized commodities, which include food grains, sugar, edible oils, kerosene, matches, and soap. Group-managed shops are more likely to be transparent, can be just as efficient as those managed by individual traders, and can assist in building up demand from the poor for better services across the board.

Women's groups could also be instrumental in rationalizing the nutrition-related programs that exist at the village level, including the ICDS and the NMMP, ensuring that households, women, and children most at risk are covered by the relevant programs. The small food supplements provided to pregnant women and children under six in the ICDS program could go a long way to ensure better nutrition and health of these vulnerable groups if combined with steady and relatively adequate food availability in their households. Currently, the ICDS program's food supplements tend to substitute for household food both at the individual and household levels. Similarly, the nutritional value of midday meals could be enhanced by targeting those most in need, such as the 3–6-year-olds who have been malnourished in early childhood and girls (and some boys) who are about to enter adolescence.

## What Must be Done and What Will It Cost?

Many of the actions needed to achieve the above objectives involve relatively little additional cost. Assigning higher priority to nutritional training; devolving responsibility to the state, district, and village levels; and fostering greater health-nutrition collaboration do not increase the cost of programs. Having a second village-level worker for health or preschool education will involve additional cost but not a very large one, especially in the context of overall spending on food and nutrition. On the other hand, expanding the ICDS or the NMMP to fully cover their target groups will require a large increase in funding. What is needed most is political will, community ownership, strong work ethic, and commitment to supplying workers with the tools they need to do their jobs.

*Political Commitment.* To reduce malnutrition in India, the most critical resource is not financial but political commitment. Malnutrition fails to receive the priority it deserves in India, as in many countries, because it is largely invisible, program efforts do not extend across many sectors and levels, and, above all, sustained political commitment is lacking for the long and difficult task of prevention. Inadequate commitment to deal with the problem effectively also manifests itself in the pervasive corruption within the programs, which results in few resources reaching the poor. It is urgently necessary to address this problem. Political commitment to improved nutrition should be demonstrated by sustained allocation and proper direction of the necessary financial and human resources. The critical needs of each of the four action areas described above, and their resource requirements, are discussed below.

*Enhancing the Quality and Impact of the ICDS.* The priority actions for the ICDS program are:

• Ensuring attention to 6–24-month-old children and pregnant women

• Enhancing quality and impact through better training, supervision, and community ownership

• Establishing a reliable monitoring and evaluation system as soon as possible

• Reducing the AWW overload and improving coverage of hamlets by either hiring a second worker or separating the preschool education component from the rest of the program

The proposed measures to decentralize the ICDS and place its management increasingly in the hands of *panchayati raj* institutions are likely to be budget-neutral in the medium term. But the extensive training that will be required immediately will mean additional resources. The Bank-financed Woman and Child Development Project could provide the necessary resources for the next five years from the US$100 million national training component. Additional resources of about US$30 million a year are required for the second worker and for the necessary quality improvements. Coverage expansion of the ICDS program should be frozen until the quality and impact of the program are satisfactory, which should be achievable within 3–5 years if sincere efforts are made. Following this, reaching all those in need nationally, i.e., the one-third of families living in poverty, would cost on the order of an additional US$250 million a year. The ICDS will therefore need an additional US$300 million per year to have a substantial impact on malnutrition.

*Household Food Security through the TPDS.* From a nutritional standpoint, the urgent priorities for the TPDS are:

• Effectively covering the poor and shifting the food subsidy entirely to the population below the poverty line

• Carefully monitoring programs to ensure benefits reach the poor

• Ensuring that the vulnerable are reached quickly with needed supplies during droughts and other disasters

When substantial improvement in the ICDS program is evident in, say, three years, 10 percent of the PDS funds should be reallocated to finance the needed expansion of the ICDS program.

*Increasing the Impact of the NMMP.* This increased impact could be achieved by two actions:

• Targeting the NMMP by area, using low educational attainment and poverty criteria

• Targeting food to preschool as well as primary school children in areas not covered by the ICDS program

These goals could be achieved without additional resources and would increase substantially the overall education and nutritional impact, and the cost-effectiveness of the program.

*Strengthening the Contribution of the Health Sector.* The priority actions needed in the health sector are:

• Training programs to ensure a quantum leap in the nutrition knowledge and capacity of all levels of health workers

• Much greater synergy with nutrition programs, especially the ICDS, and particularly by focusing the ANM–AWW collaboration on 6–24-month-olds and pregnant women

The cost would not exceed US$5 million annually, and the prospect of attracting external financing would be good.

*Rebuilding Institutional Capacity.* Rebuilding India's capacity for nutrition action, training, research, and advocacy will require:

• Constructing a high-level policy, planning, and implementation structure

• Involving *panchayati raj* institutions in a major way

• Setting clear quantitative goals and auditing them at least annually in a high-profile national conference

• Making key institutions such as the NIN and the NIPCCD autonomous and strengthening a broad network of nutrition institutions

Additional funds will be needed on a sustained basis for 10–15 years in order to assure a steady buildup of capacity to undertake the tasks outlined at the beginning of this chapter, and to provide the environment necessary to attract scientists and other professionals to careers in nutrition. Approximately US$5 million per year will be needed for the NIN and the NIPCCD, plus about US$20 million per year for 20–25 colleges of home science, medicine, or other agencies, such as the Central Food Technology Research Institute (CFTRI). The World Bank is a possible source of financial support for capacity building.

*Total Cost.* The annual total of additional resources needed is around US$80 million for a period of 10 years: a total investment of approximately US$800 million, excluding the cost of expanding the ICDS program, which could be financed by reallocating about 10 percent of the PDS budget. Since the achievement of nutrition goals is a responsibility shared among several departments, reallocation of resources across departments must be guided by their relative effectiveness in combating malnutrition. When one considers that the cost of malnutrition in lost productivity, illness, and death is at least US$10 billion annually, the cost-benefit ratio of these investments is readily apparent. Nothing less will overcome the crisis of malnutrition in India.

# Notes

1. India defines its "poverty line" in nutritional terms. It is the consumption expenditure level below which a household (of 5.5 persons on average) cannot meet the recommended intake of 2,400 calories per adult in rural areas or 2,100 in urban areas.

2. In this report, malnutrition is defined as poor nutritional status caused by some combination of low food intake, illness, and inadequate care. We include micronutrient deficiencies in the term "malnutrition" but not the problems of overnutrition (e.g., obesity), although overnutrition is increasing among the affluent in India.

3. World Bank. 1997. *India: Achievements and Challenges in Reducing Poverty.* World Bank Country Study. Washington, D.C.

4. World Bank. 1998. *India—Reducing Poverty in India: Options for More Effective Public Services.* South Asia Region, Poverty Reduction and Economic Management Division. Washington, D.C.

5. World Bank. 1998. "India—Rural Development: Options for a Growth, Poverty Oriented Fiscal Adjustment Strategy." South Asia Region, Rural Development Unit. Washington, D.C. Processed.

6. World Bank. 1998. "India—Foodgrain Marketing Policies: Reforming to Meet Food Security Needs." South Asia Region, Rural Development Unit. Washington, D.C. Processed.

7. IIPS (International Institute for Population Sciences). 1995. *National Family Health Survey (MCH and Family Planning), India 1992–93.* Bombay.

8. Indian Council of Medical Research. 1989. Evaluation of the National Nutritional Anemia Prophylaxis Programme. New Delhi.

9. IIPS (International Institute for Population Sciences). 1995. *National Family Health Survey (MCH and Family Planning), India 1992–93.* Bombay.

10. Shariff, Abusaleh, and A. C. Mallick. 1998. "Dynamics of Food Intake and Nutrition According to Income Class in India." New Delhi: National Council of Applied Economic Research. Processed.

11. Government of India. 1998b. *Annual Report 1997–98*. New Delhi: Ministry of Health and Family Welfare.

12. IIPS (International Institute for Population Sciences). 1995. *National Family Health Survey (MCH and Family Planning), India 1992–93*. Bombay.

13. ASCI (Administrative Staff College of India). 1997. *National Strategy to Reduce Childhood Malnutrition*. Hyderabad.

14. Government of India. 1997. *Focus on the Poor—Guidelines for the Implementation of the Targeted Public Distribution System*. New Delhi: Ministry of Civil Supplies, Consumer Affairs and Public Distribution.

15. Government of India. 1993. *National Nutrition Policy*. New Delhi: Department of Women and Child Development.

16. Government of India. 1995. *National Plan of Action for Nutrition*. New Delhi: Department of Women and Child Development.

17. Greene, James. 1996. "Privatizing ICDS—Problems and Prospects." Washington, D.C.: World Bank. Processed.

18. NFI. (Nutrition Foundation of India). 1988. *The Integrated Child Development Services (ICDS) Scheme*. New Delhi.

19. NIPCCD. (National Institute of Public Cooperation and Child Development). 1992. *National Evaluation of Integrated Child Development Services*. New Delhi.

20. Based on data provided by the Department of Education, Ministry of Human Resource Development, Government of India.

21. IIPS (International Institute for Population Sciences). 1995. *National Family Health Survey (MCH and Family Planning), India 1992–93*. Bombay.

22. Radhakrishna, Rokkam. 1997. "Food, Nutrition and PDS: Emerging Issues." Processed.

23.   Subbarao, Kalanidhi. 1990. *Improving Nutrition in India*. Discussion Paper No. 49. Washington, D.C.: World Bank.

24. Radhakrishna, Rokkam, and K. Subbarao. 1997. "India's Public Distribution System: A National and International Perspective." Discussion Paper No. 380. Washington, D.C.: World Bank.

25. As the relationship between these variables is complex, and data are for overlapping years, we cannot assess definitively a cause and effect relationship between levels of spending and malnutrition or poverty levels.

26. Radhakrishna, Rokkam, and K. V. Narayana. 1993. "Nutritional Programs in India: Review and Assessment." Center for Economic and Social Studies. Hyderabad.

27. World Bank. 1993. "India Public Expenditure Review, Annex IVC: Nutrition Sector." South Asia Region, Country Department II, Population and Human Resources Operations Division. Washington, D.C. Processed.

28. Government of India. 1996. National Sample Survey Organization. *Nutritional Intake in India, Fifth Quinquennial Survey on Consumer Expenditure*. New Delhi: Department of Statistics.

29. Government of India. 1998a. *Economic Survey 1997–98*. New Delhi: Ministry of Finance, Economic Division.

30. NCAER (National Council of Applied Economic Research). 1998. *Integrated Child Development Services—A Detailed Report of Pilot Study*. New Delhi.

31. Chatterjee, Meera. 1997. "Does ICDS Alleviate Poverty?" World Bank, India Country Department. New Delhi. Processed.

32. Chatterjee, Meera. "Lessons Learned from 20 Years of ICDS." 1996. World Bank, India Country Department. New Delhi. Processed.

33. World Bank. 1998. *Implementation Completion Report, India, Second Tamil Nadu Integrated Nutrition Project (Credit 2158-IN)*. World Bank, South Asia Region, Health, Nutrition and Population Sector Unit. Washington, D.C.

34. World Bank. 1998. *Implementation Completion Report, India, Integrated Child Development Services (Credit 2173-IN)*. World Bank, South Asia Region, Health, Nutrition and Population Sector Unit. Washington, D.C.

35. Radhakrishna, Rokkam, S. Indrakant, and C. Ravi. 1998. "India's Integrated Child Development Services Program: Assessments and Options for Reform." Center for Economic and Social Studies. Hyderabad.

36. Central Technical Committee. 1996. *Survey, Evaluation and Research System in Integrated Child Development Services, 1975–1995*. New Delhi.

37. Sachdev, Harsh Pal Singh. 1997. "Low Birth Weight in South Asia" in *Malnutrition in South Asia: A Regional Profile*. Stuart Gillespie, Editor. UNICEF Regional Office for South Asia, 23–50. Kathmandu.

38. Ceesay, S. M., A. M. Prentice, T. J. Cole, F. Ford, L. T. Weaver, E. M. E. Poskitt, and R. J. Whitehead. 1993. "Effects on Birth Weight and Prenatal Mortality of Maternal Dietary Supplements in Rural Gambia: 5 Year Randomized Control Trial." *British Medical Journal* 315: 786–90.

# Statistical Appendix

## List of Tables

# Table 1. Percent Prevalence of Malnutrition among Children Aged 1–4 Years in India and Selected States, 1992–93

| Country or State | Underweight (Weight-for-age below 2SD of the median) | | | Stunted (Height-for-age below 2SD of the median) | | | Wasted (Weight-height below 2SD of the median) | | |
|---|---|---|---|---|---|---|---|---|---|
| | Rural | Urban | Total | Rural | Urban | Total | Rural | Urban | Total |
| INDIA | 59.9 | 45.2 | 53.1 | 54.1 | 44.8 | 52.0 | 18.0 | 15.8 | 17.5 |
| Andhra Pradesh | 52.1 | 40. | 49.1 | — | — | — | — | — | — |
| Assam | 51.8 | 37.3 | 50.4 | 53.5 | 39.6 | 52.5 | 11.4 | 5.6 | 10.8 |
| Bihar | 64.1 | 53.8 | 62.6 | 61.8 | 55.2 | 60.9 | 22.7 | 16.3 | 21.8 |
| Gujarat | 45.8 | 40.5 | 44.1 | 44.6 | 41.6 | 43.6 | 20.3 | 16.1 | 18.9 |
| Haryana | 39.4 | 33.0 | 37.9 | 48.0 | 42.4 | 46.7 | 5.7 | 6.4 | 5.9 |
| Himachal Pradesh | 48.3 | 30.2 | 47.0 | — | — | — | — | — | — |
| Jammu-Kashmir | — | — | 44.5 | — | — | 40.8 | — | — | 14.8 |
| Karnataka | — | — | 54.3 | — | — | 47.6 | — | — | 17.4 |
| Kerala | 30.6 | 22.9 | 28.5 | 29.6 | 21.5 | 27.4 | 11.5 | 12.0 | 11.6 |
| Madhya Pradesh | 59.4 | 50.1 | 57.4 | — | — | — | — | — | — |
| Maharashtra | 57.5 | 45.5 | 52.6 | 50.8 | 39.1 | 46.0 | 21.5 | 18.3 | 20.2 |
| Orissa | — | — | 53.3 | — | — | 48.2 | — | — | 21.3 |
| Punjab | 47.4 | 40.0 | 45.9 | 40.4 | 38.4 | 40.0 | 21.4 | 14.3 | 19.9 |
| Rajasthan | 41.1 | 43.9 | 41.6 | 43.0 | 43.5 | 43.1 | 17.7 | 29.1 | 19.5 |
| Tamil Nadu | 52.1 | 37.3 | 46.6 | — | — | — | — | — | — |
| Uttar Pradesh | — | — | 49.8 | — | — | 49.2 | — | — | 16.2 |
| West Bengal | — | — | 56.8 | — | — | 43.2 | — | — | 11.9 |

— Not available.

Notes: Children below two standard deviations of the International Reference Population Median are considered malnourished.

Source: International Institute for Population Sciences. 1995. *National Family Health Survey: India, 1992–93*. Bombay.

## Table 2. Percentage Distribution Of Children Aged 1–5 Years According to Nutritional Status, Rural Areas of Selected Indian States, 1975–79, 1988–90, and 1994

| State | Period | Normal | Mild | Moderate | Severe |
|---|---|---|---|---|---|
| Andhra Pradesh | 1975–79 | 6.1 | 32.4 | 46.1 | 15.4 |
| | 1988–90 | 8.7 | 39.5 | 44.3 | 7.5 |
| | 1994 | 4.8 | 46.1 | 41.7 | 7.4 |
| Gujarat | 1975–79 | 3.8 | 28.1 | 54.3 | 13.8 |
| | 1988–90 | 7.3 | 33.9 | 45.8 | 13.0 |
| | 1994 | 4.8 | 28.0 | 55.1 | 12.1 |
| Karnataka | 1975–79 | 4.6 | 31.1 | 50.0 | 14.3 |
| | 1988–90 | 4.8 | 38.1 | 48.8 | 8.3 |
| | 1994 | 6.2 | 40.6 | 46.0 | 7.2 |
| Kerala | 1975–79 | 7.5 | 35.7 | 46.5 | 10.3 |
| | 1988–90 | 17.7 | 47.4 | 32.9 | 2.0 |
| | 1994 | 15.1 | 50.6 | 32.6 | 1.7 |
| Madhya Pradesh | 1975–79 | 8.4 | 30.3 | 45.1 | 16.2 |
| | 1988–90 | 17.7 | 27.4 | 38.9 | 16.0 |
| | 1994 | 10.2 | 36.1 | 42.1 | 11.6 |
| Maharashtra | 1975–79 | 3.2 | 25.4 | 49.5 | 21.9 |
| | 1988–90 | 6.7 | 38.0 | 47.5 | 7.8 |
| | 1994 | 8.6 | 37.2 | 43.7 | 10.5 |
| Orissa | 1975–79 | 7.5 | 35.9 | 41.7 | 14.9 |
| | 1988–90 | 8.1 | 34.6 | 46.6 | 10.7 |
| | 1994 | 6.3 | 40.4 | 47.9 | 5.4 |
| Tamil Nadu | 1975–79 | 6.2 | 34.2 | 47.0 | 12.6 |
| | 1988–90 | 8.0 | 42.0 | 45.8 | 4.2 |
| | 1994 | 13.2 | 46.7 | 36.8 | 3.3 |
| All 8 States | 1975–79 | 5.9 | 31.6 | 47.5 | 15.0 |
| | 1988–90 | 9.9 | 37.6 | 43.8 | 8.9 |
| | 1994 | 8.5 | 40.4 | 47.9 | 5.4 |

*Note*: Nutritional grades are based on NCHS (U.S. National Center for Health Statistics) Standards.

*Sources:* National Nutrition Monitoring Bureau. 1991. *Report of Repeat Survey, 1988-90*. National Institute of Nutrition. Hyderabad; and National Nutrition Monitoring Bureau. 1996. *Report for the Year 1994*. Hyderabad: National Institute of Nutrition.

## Table 3.  Percent Prevalence of Malnutrition among 1–5-Year-Old Children in India between 1975–79 and 1994

| Malnutrition Index | NNMB 1975–79 (n=6,428) | NNMB 1988–90 (n=13,422) | NNMB 1994 (n=1,832) | NFHS 1992–93 (n=25,578)[a] |
|---|---|---|---|---|
| Underweight | | | | |
| Weight for age | | | | |
| <2 SD | 77.5 | 68.6 | 63.6 | 53.4 |
| <3 SD (severe) | 38.0 | 26.6 | 24.7 | 20.6 |
| Stunting | | | | |
| Height for age | | | | |
| <2SD | 78.6 | 65.1 | 63.0 | 52.0 |
| <3SD (severe) | 53.3 | 36.8 | 35.8 | 28.9 |
| Wasting | | | | |
| Weight for height | | | | |
| <2SD | 18.1 | 19.9 | 16.7 | 17.5 |
| <3SD (severe) | 2.9 | 2.4 | 2.6 | 3.2 |

a. For weight-for-age assessment only; the sample size for the other two indices was lower.

*Source:* Sachdev, H. P. S. 1997. Nutritional Status of Children and Women in India: Recent Trends. *NFI Bulletin.* Vol.18, No. 3. p. 2.

## Table 4.  Prevalence of Malnutrition among Male and Female Children between 1 and 5 Years of Age in Ludhiana, Punjab, 1990

| Grade of Malnutrition | Females N | Females Percent | Males N | Males Percent | Relative Risk (Female/Male) |
|---|---|---|---|---|---|
| Normal | 38 | 18.3 | 72 | 35.1 | 0.52 |
| Grade I | 67 | 32.2 | 78 | 38.0 | 0.85 |
| Grade II | 59 | 28.4 | 33 | 16.1 | 1.76 |
| Grade III | 44 | 21.1 | 22 | 10.7 | 1.97 |

*Source:* Zachariah, A., and P. Zachariah 1992. The Slums of Ludhiana City (Punjab): A Case Study. *NFI Bulletin,* Vol.13, No. 2, p. 6.

## Table 5.   Percentage Distribution of Adult Women by Body Mass Index in India between 1975–79 and 1994

| | Body Mass Index | NNMB Rural 1975-79 (n=6,428) | NNMB Rural 1988-90 (n=13,422) | NNMB Rural 1994 (n=1,832) | NNMB Urban 1993-94 (n=1,319) |
|---|---|---|---|---|---|
| Chronically Energy-deficient | | | | | |
| Third degree | <16 | 12.7 | 11.3 | 10.4 | 9.5 |
| Second degree | 16-17 | 13.2 | 12.9 | 11.2 | 9.2 |
| First degree | 17-18.5 | 25.9 | 25.1 | 25.5 | 18.0 |
| All | <18.5 | 51.8 | 49.3 | 47.1 | 36.7 |
| Normal | 18.5-25 | 44.9 | 46.6 | 46.3 | 51.7 |
| Obese | >25 | 3.4 | 4.1 | 6.6 | 11.6 |

*Note*: Body Mass Index (BMI) is defined as weight (Kg)/ Height$^2$ (m).
*Source*: Sachdev, H. P. S.  1997. Nutritional Status of Children and Women in India: Recent Trends. *NFI Bulletin*  Vol.18,  No. 3, p. 3.


## Table 6.   Mean Birth Weights of Infants in Different Regions of India and Proportion of Low Birth Weight, 1990

| Study Center | Mean Birth Weight grams | Birth Weight below 2,500 gm. percent |
|---|---|---|
| Delhi | 2764 + 545 | 25.1 |
| Varanasi | 2628 + 504 | 30.6 |
| Madras | 2710 + 536 | 23.0 |
| Trivandrum | 2881 + 533 | 15.3 |
| Calcutta | 2673 + 394 | 20.1 |
| Jamshedpur | 2693 + 437 | 19.0 |
| Baroda | 2449 + 520 | 46.4 |
| Bombay | 2597 + 441 | 34.9 |
| Asia (1990) | — | 21 |
| Africa (1990) | — | 15 |
| Developing Countries (1990) | — | 19 |
| Developed Countries (1990) | — | 7 |
| Global (1990) | — | 17 |

—Not available

*Source*: Ramachandran, P. 1993. Low Birth Weights: The Indian Experience. *NFI Bulletin* Vol. 14,  No. 4. p. 5.

## Table 7.   Recent Trends in Prevalence Of Low Birth Weight in India, Various Years

| Area | Setting | Comparison period (mean) gap in years) | Change in Birth Weight | Change in Gestation | Change in IUG |
|------|---------|----------------------------------------|------------------------|---------------------|---------------|
| Rourkela, Orissa | Industrial hospital | 1963 & 1986 (23) | MBW+74g. LBW: 34 vs. 24 percent | | — |
| Delhi | Hospital (poor) | 1969 & 1989 (20) | — | Term | 0 |
| Delhi | Hospital (better off) | 1973-4 & 1985-7 (13) | — | — | + |
| North Arcot, Tamil Nadu | Rural | 1969-73 & 1989-93 (20) | MBW+78g. LBW: 27 vs. 16 percent | M+0.7W PTL 21 vs. 16 percent | +p |
| | Urban | 1969-73 & 1989-93 (20) | MBW+52g. LBW: 19 vs. 11 percent | M+0.8W PT: 20 vs. 15 percent | +p |
| Vellore | Hospital | 1969 & 1994 (25) | MBW+126g. LBW: 27 vs. 15 percent | Me+0.3W PT: 14 vs. 10 percent | — |
| Mumbai | Hospital (poor) | 1988 & 1995 (8) | LBW: 60 vs. 38 percent | 0 | — |
| Delhi | Hospital (poor) | 1986 & 14996 (10) | 0 | 0 | — |

Notes: + = significant increase; +p = significant increase at some gestations;   0 =  no significant change; IUG = Intrauterine growth; M = Mean;  Me = median;  MBW = mean birth weight;  W = gestational weeks; — Not available.

Source. Sachdev, H.P.S. 1997.  Low Birth Weight in South Asia in *Malnutrition in South Asia: A Regional Profile.* p. 31. Kathmandu: UNICEF.

## Table 8.  Prevalence of Anemia among Pregnant Women in Selected States of India, Various Years

| | Percent of Women with Hemoglobin | |
| | below 11 grams | below 8 grams |
| State | per deciliter | per deciliter |
|---|---|---|
| Andhra Pradesh | 47.0 | 14.0 |
| Bihar | 81.0 | — |
| Delhi | 61.0 | — |
| Gujarat | 84.0 | 21.0 |
| Haryana | 95.0 | — |
| Maharashtra | 87.0 | 41.0 |
| Rajasthan | 98.0 | — |
| Tamil Nadu | 54.0 | — |
| Uttar Pradesh | 80.0 | — |

— Not available.

*Source:* Government of India 1996. *Report of the Task Force on Micronutrients (Vitamin A and Iron).* New Delhi: Ministry of Human Resource Development, Department of Women and Child Development.

## Table 9.  Prevalence of Anemia among Lactating Women in Selected Urban Areas of India, Various Years

| | Percent of Women with Hemoglobin | |
| | below 12 grams | below 8 grams |
| Location | per deciliter | per deciliter |
|---|---|---|
| Baroda | 77.0 | 13.0 |
| Bombay | 90.0 | 10.0 |
| Calcutta | 95.0 | 15.0 |
| Madras | 81.0 | 14.0 |

*Source:* Government of India 1996. *Report of the Task Force on Micronutrients (Vitamin A and Iron).* New Delhi: Ministry of Human Resource Development, Department of Women and Child Development.

## Table 10. Prevalence of Anemia among Preschool Children in Various Locations in India, Various Years

| | Percent of Children with Hemoglobin | |
| | below 11 grams | below 7 grams |
| Location | per deciliter | per deciliter |
| --- | --- | --- |
| Andhra Pradesh (Hyderabad) | 64 | 6 |
| Delhi | 72 | — |
| Gujarat (Baroda) | 67 | 6 |
| Maharashtra (Bombay & Pune) | 48 | — |
| Tamil Nadu (Vellore & Madras) | 30 | — |
| Uttar Pradesh (Varanasi) | 63 | — |
| West Bengal (Calcutta) | 95 | 18 |

— Not available.

*Source:* Government of India 1996. *Report of the Task Force on Micronutrients (Vitamin A and Iron).* New Delhi: Ministry of Human Resource Development, Department of Women and Child Development.

## Table 11. Percent Prevalence of Anemia among Different Age and Sex Groups in Rural Locations of India, 1981

| Age (years) | Sex | Hyderabad | Delhi | Calcutta |
| --- | --- | --- | --- | --- |
| 1-5 | M+F | 65.9 | 59.0 | 95.4 |
| 6-14 | M | 55.0 | 72.4 | 96.1 |
| | F | 65.3 | 69.4 | 97.0 |
| 15-22 | M | 38.7 | 65.1 | 90.1 |
| | F | 69.2 | 63.7 | 96.7 |
| 25-44 | M | 80.1 | 57.3 | 88.6 |
| | F | 71.4 | 71.3 | 96.4 |
| >45 | M+F | 47.6 | 59.3 | 92.4 |

*Source:* Narasinga Rao, B.S. 1991. Prevention and Control of Anemia in India: Theory and Practice. *NFI Bulletin.* Vol. 12, No. 2. p. 4.

## Table 12.  Prevalence of Vitamin A Deficiency in Preschoolers between 1965-69 and 1994

| Survey | Period | Percent |
|---|---|---|
| ICMR | 1965-69 | 4.2 |
| NNMB 1975-79 | 1975-79 | 1.8 |
| NNMB 1988-90 | 1988-90 | 0.7 |
| NNMB 1992-93[a] | 1992-93 | 1.9 |
| NNMB 1994 | 1994 | 1.1 |
| NNMB Slum[b] | 1993-94 | 0.9 to 2.5 |

*Notes:* Vitamin A deficiency was estimated on the basis of the presence of Bitot's spots.
a. This survey included two additional states (Uttar Pradesh and West Bengal) that were not in other NNMB surveys.
b. Data from only three of six cities that were surveyed.
*Source*: Sachdev, H. P. S. (1997). Nutritional Status of Children and Women in India: Recent Trends. *NFI Bulletin*. Vol.18,  No. 3, p. 4.

## Table 13.  Percent Prevalence of Goitre among Males and Females in Various Districts of India, 1984-86

| Districts | All Persons | Male | Female | Ratio (F/M) |
|---|---|---|---|---|
| Visakhapatnam, Andhra Pradesh | 15.8 | 7.0 | 24.6 | 3.5 |
| Dibrugarh, Assam | 65.8 | 51.4 | 77.6 | 1.5 |
| Muzaffarpur, Bihar | 33.8 | 29.8 | 36.9 | 1.2 |
| Sitamari, Bihar | 31.8 | 27.6 | 35.4 | 1.3 |
| Surat, Gujarat | 22.7 | 14.6 | 29.7 | 2.0 |
| Mandla, Gujarat | 34.4 | 29.9 | 39.4 | 1.3 |
| Dhule, Maharashtra | 16.5 | 11.6 | 20.9 | 1.8 |
| Central Manipur | 10.4 | 5.2 | 15.7 | 3.0 |
| West Manipur | 19.8 | 14.8 | 23.7 | 1.6 |
| Nilgiri, Tamil Nadu | 6.9 | 2.9 | 10.5 | 3.6 |
| Bahraich, Uttar Pradesh | 20.2 | 18.0 | 22.5 | 1.3 |
| Basti, Uttar Pradesh | 20.0 | 16.0 | 24.3 | 1.5 |
| Gorakhpur, Uttar Pradesh | 18.6 | 12.2 | 26.2 | 2.1 |
| Mirzapur, Uttar Pradesh | 6.2 | 3.9 | 8.9 | 2.3 |
| All 14 Districts | 21.1 | 15.5 | 26.8 | 1.7 |

*Source*:  Indian Council of Medical Research (1989). *Epidemiological Survey of Endemic Goitre and Endemic Cretinism: An ICMR Task Force Study*. p. 29. New Delhi.

## Table 14.  Proportion of 6-9 Month-Old Infants Receiving Breast Milk and Solid Foods,  India and Selected States, 1992-93

| State | Percent |
|-------|---------|
| INDIA | 31.4 |
| Andhra Pradesh | 47.8 |
| Assam | 39.2 |
| Bihar | 18.1 |
| Gujarat | 22.9 |
| Karnataka | 38.2 |
| Kerala | 69.3 |
| Madhya Pradesh | 27.7 |
| Maharashtra | 25.0 |
| Orissa | 30.2 |
| Rajasthan | 9.4 |
| Tamil Nadu | 56.5 |
| Uttar Pradesh | 19.4 |
| West Bengal | 53.6 |

*Source*: International Institute for Population Sciences. 1995. *National Family Health Survey, 1992-93*.  Bombay.

**Table 15. Average Nutrient Intake of Children and Adults as a Percentage of Recommended Dietary Intakes in India, 1988-90**

| | Protein | Energy | Calcium | Iron | Vitamin A | Thiamin | Riboflavin | Niacin | Vitamin C |
|---|---|---|---|---|---|---|---|---|---|
| Children | | | | | | | | | |
| 1-3 yrs | 94.5 | 62.8 | 61.2 | 71.7 | 35.2 | 66.7 | 51.4 | 60.0 | 48.3 |
| 7-9 yrs | 90.7 | 71.8 | 92.7 | 67.7 | 34.8 | 82.0 | 46.7 | 70.0 | 44.8 |
| Adolescents (13-15 yrs) | | | | | | | | | |
| Boys | 72.0 | 81.3 | 71.8 | 58.3 | 48.0 | 87.5 | 47.3 | 78.1 | 94.5 |
| Girls | 74.9 | 91.8 | 65.8 | 78.6 | 37.8 | 101.0 | 58.3 | 87.1 | 75.2 |
| Adults | | | | | | | | | |
| Males | 108.0 | 87.5 | 144.2 | 109.6 | 48.5 | 100.0 | 73.7 | 90.5 | 101.0 |
| Females | | | | | | | | | |
| NPNL [a] | 108.0 | 90.6 | 113.7 | 87.3 | 40.5 | 103.6 | 56.9 | 93.6 | 81.2 |
| Pregnant | 65.0 | 75.6 | 48.3 | 35.5 | 63.0 | 89.1 | 53.0 | 80.0 | 91.0 |
| Lactating | 75.2 | 89.1 | 51.5 | 87.0 | 32.9 | 103.0 | 59.3 | 90.0 | 47.5 |

a. NPNL = Non-Pregnant and Non-Lactating.
Source: Bamji, M., and A. V. Lakshmi (1993). Less Recognized Micronutrient Deficiencies in India. *NFI Bulletin.* Vol. 19, No. 2. p. 5.

## Table 16.  Caloric Intake of Preschool Children, by Nutritional Status, in India, 1975-79 and 1988-90

| Nutritional Status | Caloric Intake (kcal./day) | |
|---|---|---|
| (percent of weight for age)[a] | 1975-79 | 1988-90 |
| > 90  (Normal) | 1035 | 1013 |
| 90-75  (Mild) | 995 | 988 |
| 75-60  (Moderate) | 884 | 928 |
| < 60  (Severe) | 812 | 796 |

a. NCHS (U.S. National Center  of Health Statistics) Standards.

*Source:*  National Nutrition Monitoring Bureau (1991). *Report of Repeat Surveys  (1988-90).* Hyderabad: National Institute of Nutrition.


## Table 17.  Per Capita Consumption Expenditure and Nutrient Intake of the Poorest 30 Percent of the Population of India in 1972–73 and 1987–88 (at 1987–88 prices; Indian Rupees per month)

|  | Rural | | | Urban | | |
|---|---|---|---|---|---|---|
|  | 1972-73 | 1987-88 | Percent change | 1972-73 | 1987-88 | Percent change |
| Commodity | | | | | | |
| Cereal & cereal substitutes | 16.41 | 16.50 | 0.55 | 15.59 | 16.36 | 4.94 |
| Non-cereal food | 8.87 | 12.71 | 43.29 | 15.17 | 21.25 | 40.08 |
| All food | 25.28 | 29.21 | 15.55 | 30.76 | 37.61 | 22.27 |
| Non-food | 6.98 | 11.19 | 60.32 | 10.81 | 16.19 | 29.42 |
| Total Expenditure | 32.26 | 40.40 | 25.23 | 41.57 | 53.80 | 29.42 |
| | | | | | | |
| Nutrient Intake | | | | | | |
| Calories (Kcal/day) | 1,510 | 1,599 | 5.89 | 1,524 | 1,704 | 11.81 |
| Protein (g./day) | 41.25 | 42.98 | 4.19 | 40.23 | 46.00 | 14.34 |

*Source*: R. Radhakrishna and C. Ravi (1996) cited in R. Radhakrishna (1997). *Food, Nutrition and PDS: Emerging Issues.* Indian Econometric Society, University of Hyderabad. Processed.

**Table 18. Foodgrain Production and Availability in India for Various Years between 1951 and 1995**

| | Net production (metric tons) | Imports (metric tons) | Total availability (metric tons) | Per capita availability (grams/day) | | PDS (metric tons) | |
|---|---|---|---|---|---|---|---|
| | | | | Total | From domestic production | Procurement | Off take |
| 1951 | 48.1 | 4.8 | 52.4 | 395 | 363 | 3.8 | 8.0 |
| 1961 | 72.0 | 3.5 | 75.7 | 469 | 446 | 0.5 | 4.0 |
| 1971 | 94.4 | 2.0 | 94.3 | 469 | 472 | 8.9 | 7.8 |
| 1981 | 113.4 | 0.7 | 114.3 | 455 | 451 | 13.0 | 13.0 |
| 1991 | 154.3 | -0.1 | 158.6 | 510 | 496 | 19.6 | 20.8 |
| 1995 | 167.2 | — | 167.8 | 502 | 500 | 22.5 | 15.3 |

— Not available.

*Note:* Total availability = Net Production + Imports – Changes in Government stocks.

*Source:* Government of India (1997). *Economic Survey, 1995-96.* New Delhi.

## Table 19. Usage of Iron Folic Acid by Pregnant Woman Who Received the Tablets, by Selected Characteristics, Uttar Pradesh, 1995-96

| Characteristics | Number of cases | Percent of Women who | | |
| --- | --- | --- | --- | --- |
| | | Used all | Partially used | Not used at all |
| Age | | | | |
|   Less than 25 years | 39 | 36 | 49 | 15 |
|   25-29 years | 52 | 52 | 39 | 10 |
|   30+ years | 26 | 39 | 42 | 19 |
| Pregnancy | | | | |
|   1 | 33 | 39 | 49 | 12 |
|   2+ | 88 | 46 | 40 | 15 |
| Number of tablets supplied[a] | | | | |
|   25-50 tablets | 41 | 24 | 56 | 20 |
|   51-75 tablets | 20 | 45 | 55 | — |
|   100 + tablets | 60 | 57 | 28 | 15 |
| Knew the benefits of iron | | | | |
|   Yes | 63 | 62 | 37 | 2 |
|   No | 58 | 24 | 48 | 28 |

a. Indicates significance at 1 percent level.
*Source*: Tuladhar, J. M. and others (1997). Iron Supplementation: Knowledge, Perceptions and Usage Among Pregnant Women in Rural India. Technical Paper 9. p. 8. New Delhi: Population Council.

**Table 20.  Percentage Distribution by Nutritional Status of 0-36 Month-Old Children in the World Bank-Assisted Tamil Nadu Integrated Nutrition Project Between 1992-93 and 1997**

| Data Source and Date | Normal | Grade I | Grade II | Grades III & IV |
|---|---|---|---|---|
| Baseline (Phase I-III) survey (1992-93)[a] | 41.4 | 34.9 | 18.8 | 4.9 |
| National Family Health Survey (1992-93) | 43.8 | 33.0 | 19.1 | 4.1 |
| Baseline (Phase IV and V) survey (1995) | 54.6 | 29.6 | 13.1 | 2.8 |
| Monitoring Data (December 1995) | 40.0 | 39.4 | 16.8 | 3.8 |
| Mid-term Survey (April/May 1996) | 44.7 | 26.5 | 19.0 | 9.8 |
| Monitoring Data (April 1996) | 43.8 | 40.7 | 14.3 | 1.2 |
| Monitoring Data (December 1996) | 45.4 | 40.0 | 13.5 | 1.1 |
| Terminal evaluation (October 1997)[b] | 81.8 | | 15.1 | 3.1 |

*Notes:* a. The age group for the 1992-93 baseline and 1997 endline surveys was 6–36 months,  which would be expected to give slightly higher figures than the 0-36 month aggregate.

b. The Terminal Evaluation figures refer to 9 districts for which data were available at the time of preparation of the Implementation Completion Report. The figure under *Normal* includes Grade I.

*Source*:  World Bank (1998). *Implementation Completion Report, India: Second Tamil Nadu Integrated Nutrition Project.*  Report No. 17755.  p. 4. Washington D.C.

## Table 21.  Percentage of 0–36-Month-Old Children Severely Malnourished in Different Districts of Tamil Nadu, 1996 and 1997

| District | Midterm Survey 1996 | | Terminal Evaluation 1997 | |
|---|---|---|---|---|
| | Grade II | Grades III & IV | Grade II | Grades III &IV |
| Villupuram | — | 16.1 | — | 6.0 |
| Tiruvannamalai | 24.0 | 17.4 | 13.3 | 3.3 |
| Salem | 22.4 | 12.6 | 14.4 | 2.9 |
| Dindigul | 20.5 | 11.2 | 13.9 | 3.5 |
| Madurai | 20.5 | 20.5 | 15.7 | — |
| Dharmapuri | 21.1 | — | 10.9 | — |

— Not available.

*Note*: The age group for the Terminal Evaluation was 6–36 months, which would be expected to give slightly higher figures than the 0–36 month aggregate.

*Source*: World Bank 1998. *Implementation Completion Report, India: Second Tamil Nadu Integrated Nutrition Project*. Report No. 17755. Appendix B, p. 2. Washington, D.C.

**Table 22.  Progress of Key Indicators for Project Implementation of the First World Bank-Assisted Integrated Child Development Services (ICDS) Project in Andhra Pradesh and Orissa, 1996**

| Key Implementation Indicators | Andhra Pradesh | | Orissa | |
|---|---|---|---|---|
| | Estimated percent (SAR target) | Actual percent (1996 MTS) | Estimated percent (SAR target) | Actual percent (1996MTS) |
| *Impact Indicators* | | | | |
| Reduce severe malnutrition (Grades III & IV) among children 6-36 months | 50 | 46 | 50 | 44 |
| Increase proportion of children 6-36 months in Normal and Grade 1 | 25 | 31 | 25 | 0.4 |
| Reduction in Infant Mortality Rate | 70/1000 | 66/1000 | 100/1000 | 95/1000 |
| Reduction in incidence of low birth weight | 30 | 23 | 20 | 23 |
| *Process Indicators* | | | | |
| Early registration of pregnant women | 50 | 38 | 50 | 29 |
| Total registration of pregnant women | 80 | 79 | 80 | 71 |
| Obstetrical and nutritional risk assessment of those registered | 100 | 79 | 100 | 61 |
| Tetanus toxoid immunization of pregnant women | 90 | 86 | 80 | 71 |
| Consumption of iron and folic acid tablets for at least 12 weeks by pregnant women | 60 | 8 | 60 | 15 |
| Administration of postpartum vitamin A to attended deliveries | 80 | — | 80 | — |
| Food supplement for at least 20 weeks to registered pregnant women with inadequate nutritional status | 80 | 28[a] | 60 | 26[a] |
| Food supplement for at least 16 weeks of registered lactating women with malnutrition in pregnancy | 90 | 27[a] | 90 | 23[a] |
| Immunization (UIP-6) of children | 90 | 26 | 85 | 21 |

| | | | | |
|---|---|---|---|---|
| Vitamin A megadose (100,000-200,000 i.u.) semiannually to children 6-36 months | 80 | 8 | 80 | 8 |
| Regular growth monitoring (>9 times a year) of children 0-3 years | 80 | 1 | 80 | 2 |
| Supplementation of monitored children 0-3 years with grade II-IV malnutrition | 90 | 41[a] | 90 | 42[a] |
| Completed referral of severely malnourished children ( Grades III and IV) or non-responding children 0-3 years to VHN/MPWF and PHC | 80 | — | 80 | — |
| Quarterly growth monitoring, weighing and charting of children 3-5 years (>3 times a year) | 80 | 17 | 60 | 25 |
| Referral of severely malnourished 3–5-year-old children to MPWF/PHC | 90 | — | 90 | — |
| Administration of vitamin A megadose semiannually to 3—5-year-old children | 80 | — | 70 | 7 |
| Preschool attendance (>80 % of working days) | 80 | 53 | 60 | 43 |
| Routine deparasitization of monitored children in heavily infected communities as determined by parasite surveys | 90 | — | 80 | — |
| Household use of oral rehydration in the last incidence of diarrhea in the target group | 60 | 33 | 50 | 32 |
| Treatment of pneumonia by MPWF/AWW with co-trimaxazole in cases of acute respiratory infections (ARI) | 30 | 5 | 20 | 10 |
| Additional feeds of local weaning food initiated by 6 months in infants | 60 | 47 | 50 | 48 |
| Provision of 4 additional weaning feeds/day by 9 months in infants | 60 | — | 50 | — |
| Active women's groups (>9 meetings a year) | 80 | — | 70 | — |

— Not available.

*Notes:* SAR = Staff Appraisal Report; MTS = Midterm Survey; a. Data not disaggregated by nutritional status.
*Source:* World Bank 1998. *Implementation Completion Report: India: Integrated Child Development Services Project.*. Report No: 17756. Washington D.C.

### Table 23. Percentage Distribution by Nutritional Status of 0–3-Year-Old Children in the First World Bank-Assisted ICDS Project in Andhra Pradesh and Orissa, 1990 to 1997

| Grade | 1990 | 1991 | 1992 | 1993 | 1994 | 1995 | 1996 | 1996 | 1997 |
|---|---|---|---|---|---|---|---|---|---|
| Andhra Pradesh | | | | | | | | | |
| Normal & I | 62.8 | 60.5 | 68.3 | 69.6 | 70.8 | 73.6 | 75.6 | 82.0 | 78.6 |
| II | 27.2 | 31.9 | 26.6 | 26.4 | 26.6 | 24.4 | 22.8 | 12.6 | — |
| III & IV | 10.0 | 7.6 | 5.1 | 4.0 | 2.6 | 2.0 | 1.6 | 5.4 | 5.0 |
| Orissa | | | | | | | | | |
| Normal & I | 68.4 | — | — | — | 67.8 | 69.1 | 68.9 | 68.7 | 85.5 |
| II | 23.4 | — | — | — | 26.7 | 25.9 | 26.6 | 19.5 | — |
| III & IV | 8.2 | — | — | — | 5.5 | 5.0 | 4.5 | 11.8 | 4.1 |

— Not available.

Note: Grades of malnutrition are according to the Indian Academy of Pediatrics weight-for-age classification. The figures for 1990 were based on the project Baseline Survey, and those in the second column for 1996 on the Midterm survey. The figures for 1997 are the target set by the project and derived by applying the impact objective target to the actual values.

Source: World Bank 1998. *Implementation Completion Report: India: Integrated Child Development Services Project.* Report No: 17756. Washington D.C.

### Table 24. Estimated Cost of the ICDS Program in One Project Block, Andhra Pradesh, 1996

| | Thousands of Rupees | Percentage of Total Cost |
|---|---|---|
| Health | 142.18 | 3.19 |
| Salaries | 102.78 | 2.31 |
| Traveling Allowance & Petrol | 9.40 | 0.21 |
| Medical Kits | 30.00 | 0.67 |
| Welfare | 1215.20 | 27.30 |
| Salaries | 990.60 | 22.26 |
| Wages | 3.60 | 0.08 |
| Rents | 34.86 | 0.78 |
| Traveling Allowance | 141.68 | 3.18 |
| Nutrition | | |
| Ready to Eat Food | 3093.60[a] | 69.50 |
| Total Cost | 4450.98 | 100.00 |

a. Includes transport costs.

Source: R. Radhakrishna and others. 1997. *India's Public Distribution System: A National and International Perspective.* p. 13. Washington D.C.: World Bank.

## Table 25.  Cost of Various Poverty Alleviation Programs per Rupee of Income Transferred, India, 1988-90

| Program | Cost in Rupees |
|---|---|
| Integrated Child Development Services | 1.80 |
| Maharashtra Employment Guarantee Scheme | 3.10 |
| Jawahar Rozgar Yojana | 4.35 |
| Public Distribution System | 5.37 |
| Andhra Pradesh Rice Scheme | 6.35 |

Source: R. Radhakrishna and others. 1997. India's Public Distribution System: A National and International Perspective. p. 55. Washington D.C.: World Bank.

## Table 26.  Government of India Expenditures on Food Subsidies for Various Years between 1974-75 and 1994-95

| Year | At current prices | At 1980-81 prices | Expenditure as a percent of | |
|---|---|---|---|---|
| | Indian Rupees, millions | | GNP | Total Government expenditure |
| 1974-75 | 2950 | 4238 | 0.44 | 3.01 |
| 1979-80 | 6000 | 6689 | 0.58 | 3.24 |
| 1984-85 | 11000 | 7927 | 0.53 | 2.51 |
| 1989-90 | 24760 | 12172 | 0.61 | 2.60 |
| 1994-95 | 51000 | 14920 | 0.61 | 3.01 |

Source: R. Radhakrishna and others. 1997. India's Public Distribution System: A National and International Perspective. p. 17. Washington D.C.: World Bank.

**Table 27.   Expenditure per Child Aged 0-14 Years on Supplementary Nutrition Programs in Selected States of India at Current Prices, 1990-91 to 1992-93**

| State | Severe malnutrition among 1–5-year-olds in 1988-90 (percent) | 1990-91 | 1991- 92 | 1992 – 93 |
|---|---|---|---|---|
| | | | (Indian Rupees) | |
| Andhra Pradesh | 7.5 | | | |
| Total (Center + State) | | 5.18 | 8.47 | 8.08 |
| Center | | 0.74 | 2.01 | 1.76 |
| Assam | — | | | |
| Total (Center + State) | | 1.96 | 8.03 | 9.11 |
| Center | | 1.08 | 0.10 | 2.75 |
| Haryana | — | | | |
| Total (Center  + State) | | 14.96 | 20.50 | 25.81 |
| Center | | 1.16 | 1.29 | 1.12 |
| Madhya Pradesh | 16.0 | | | |
| Total (Center  + State) | | 2.35 | 6.67 | 9.38 |
| Center | | 0.08 | 1.14 | 1.13 |
| Tamil Nadu | 4.2 | | | |
| Total (Center  + State) | | 68.65 | 162.91 | 175.94 |
| Center | | 5.64 | 6.94 | 7.31 |

Source: R. Radhakrishna and K. V. Narayana. 1993. Nutrition Programs in India: Review and Assessment. Center for Economic and Social Studies. Hyderabad. Processed.

## Table 28. Nutrition Expenditure per Malnourished Child in Selected States of India, 1993-94

| State | Number of 0–6 year-old children (millions) | Percent of children malnourished in 1992-93 | Number of malnourished children in 1992-93 (millions) | Total expenditure in 1992-93 (Rupees million) | Expenditure per malnourished child (Rupees) |
|---|---|---|---|---|---|
| Andhra Pradesh | 11 | 49.1 | 5.4 | 444 | 82.21 |
| Assam | 4 | 50.4 | 2.0 | 148 | 73.41 |
| Bihar | 18 | 62.6 | 11.3 | — | — |
| Gujarat | 7 | 44.1 | 3.1 | 902 | 292.19 |
| Haryana | 3 | 37.9 | 1.1 | 206 | 181.18 |
| Karnataka | 7 | 54.3 | 3.8 | 133 | 34.99 |
| Kerala | 3 | 28.5 | 0.9 | 156 | 182.46 |
| Madhya Pradesh | 13 | 57.4 | 7.5 | 344 | 46.10 |
| Maharashtra | 14 | 52.6 | 7.4 | 801 | 108.77 |
| Orissa | 5 | 53.3 | 2.7 | 361 | 135.46 |
| Punjab | 3 | 45.9 | 1.4 | — | — |
| Rajasthan | 9 | 41.6 | 3.7 | 167 | 44.60 |
| Tamil Nadu | 7 | 46.6 | 3.3 | 2389 | 732.37 |
| Uttar Pradesh | 29 | 49.8 | 14.4 | — | — |
| West Bengal | 12 | 56.8 | 6.8 | 244 | 35.80 |
| All 12 States | 95 | 50.0 | 47.6 | 6294 | 132.20 |

— Not available

*Notes:* The numbers of children aged 0-6 years were estimated from data from the Registrar General of India for the given years. Data on the percent of malnourished children are from the National Family Health Survey, 1992-93, which pertain to 1–4-year-olds. Rates of malnutrition among 0–6-year-olds are assumed to be similar. Children below two Standard Deviations from the International Reference Population median are considered malnourished.

*Source:* Radhakrishna, R., S. Indrakant and C. Ravi. 1998. India's Integrated Child Development Services Program – Assessment and Options for Reform. Center for Economic and Social Studies. Hyderabad. Processed.

**Table 29. Nutrition Expenditure in Selected States of India, 1990-91 to 1994-95 at Current and Constant 1994 Prices**

| State | Current prices (Indian Rupees, million) | | | | | Constant prices (1994) (Indian Rupees, million) | | | | |
|---|---|---|---|---|---|---|---|---|---|---|
| | 90-91 | 91-92 | 92-93 | 93-94 | 94-95 | 90-91 | 91-92 | 92-93 | 93-94 | 94-95 |
| Andhra Pradesh | 116 | 444 | 442 | 499 | 627 | 185 | 606 | 569 | 569 | 627 |
| Assam | 150 | 148 | 129 | 143 | 238 | 179 | 164 | 140 | 151 | 238 |
| Gujarat | 661 | 902 | 1046 | 1163 | 1358 | 981 | 1143 | 1280 | 1252 | 1358 |
| Haryana | 203 | 206 | 260 | 305 | 341 | 313 | 271 | 325 | 337 | 341 |
| Karnataka | 131 | 133 | 223 | 273 | 381 | 187 | 166 | 260 | 298 | 381 |
| Kerala | 146 | 156 | 171 | 182 | 272 | 203 | 177 | 183 | 189 | 272 |
| Madhya Pradesh | 300 | 344 | 632 | 611 | 749 | 422 | 427 | 755 | 659 | 749 |
| Maharashtra | 551 | 801 | 646 | 777 | 928 | 815 | 1045 | 776 | 858 | 928 |
| Orissa | 169 | 361 | 425 | 511 | 634 | 248 | 461 | 497 | 555 | 634 |
| Rajasthan | 141 | 167 | 204 | 280 | 307 | 185 | 183 | 213 | 268 | 307 |
| Tamil Nadu | 2327 | 2389 | 2387 | 2372 | 3025 | 2514 | 3164 | 2838 | 2561 | 3025 |
| West Bengal | 213 | 244 | 286 | 386 | 402 | 268 | 284 | 321 | 392 | 402 |
| All 12 States | 5107 | 6294 | 6849 | 7503 | 9261 | 7500 | 8092 | 8158 | 8090 | 9261 |

*Note:* Expenditure on nutrition includes central and state governments' revenue expenditure on centrally sponsored schemes, and state governments' revenue expenditure.

*Source:* Radhakrishna, R., S. Indrakant and C. Ravi. 1998. India's Integrated Child Development Services Program—Assessment and Options for Reform. Center for Economic and Social Studies. Hyderabad. Processed.

**Table 30. Nutrition Expenditures of Indian States as Percentages of the State's Total Expenditure and State Domestic Product, 1990-91 to 1994-95**

| State | Percent of State's total expenditure | | | | | Percent of State's domestic product | | | | |
|---|---|---|---|---|---|---|---|---|---|---|
| | 90-91 | 91-92 | 92-93 | 93-94 | 94-95 | 90-91 | 91-92 | 92-93 | 93-94 | 94-95 |
| Andhra Pradesh | 0.18 | 0.57 | 0.49 | 0.47 | 0.56 | 0.04 | 0.12 | 0.11 | 0.10 | 0.11 |
| Assam | 0.56 | 0.53 | 0.41 | 0.40 | 0.58 | 0.16 | 0.14 | 0.11 | 0.12 | 0.17 |
| Gujarat | 1.21 | 1.31 | 1.31 | 1.38 | 1.45 | 0.27 | 0.34 | 0.31 | 0.31 | 0.29 |
| Haryana | 0.85 | 0.75 | 0.88 | 0.74 | 0.43 | 0.17 | 0.14 | 0.17 | 0.17 | 0.16 |
| Karnataka | 0.26 | 0.21 | 0.31 | 0.34 | 0.41 | 0.06 | 0.05 | 0.08 | 0.08 | 0.10 |
| Kerala | 0.43 | 0.39 | 0.39 | 0.35 | 0.44 | 0.12 | 0.10 | 0.10 | 0.09 | 0.12 |
| Madhya Pradesh | 0.51 | 0.52 | 0.83 | 0.69 | 0.75 | 0.11 | 0.12 | 0.20 | 0.16 | 0.18 |
| Maharashtra | 0.51 | 0.66 | 0.46 | 0.49 | 0.47 | 0.10 | 0.12 | 0.08 | 0.08 | 0.08 |
| Orissa | 0.55 | 0.99 | 1.08 | 1.15 | 1.15 | 0.17 | 0.29 | 0.32 | 0.33 | 0.36 |
| Rajasthan | 0.30 | 0.29 | 0.32 | 0.38 | 0.36 | 0.08 | 0.09 | 0.09 | 0.12 | 0.13 |
| Tamil Nadu | 3.51 | 2.49 | 2.45 | 2.36 | 2.91 | 0.83 | 0.72 | 0.62 | 0.53 | 0.58 |
| West Bengal | 0.35 | 0.39 | 0.43 | 0.48 | 0.40 | 0.07 | 0.07 | 0.07 | 0.08 | 0.08 |
| All 12 States | 0.60 | 0.63 | 0.62 | 0.60 | 0.63 | 0.14 | 0.15 | 0.14 | 0.13 | 0.15 |

Source: Radhakrishna, R., S. Indrakant, and C. Ravi. 1998. India's Integrated Child Development Services Program—Assessment and Options for Reform. Center for Economic and Social Studies. Hyderabad. Processed.

**Table 31. Nutrition Expenditure per Child in Selected States of India and Annual Growth Rate (AGR) of Expenditure, 1990–91 to 1994–95**

| States | Expenditure (Indian Rupees, million) | | | | | |
|---|---|---|---|---|---|---|
|  | 90-91 | 91-92 | 92-93 | 93-94 | 94-95 | AGR |
| Current Prices |  |  |  |  |  |  |
| Andhra Pradesh | 10.54 | 39.61 | 38.82 | 43.06 | 53.26 | 2.52 |
| Assam | 33.31 | 32.17 | 27.48 | 30.03 | 48.79 | 3.29 |
| Gujarat | 95.44 | 127.77 | 145.24 | 158.47 | 181.37 | 4.48 |
| Haryana | 63.06 | 62.55 | 77.10 | 88.45 | 96.54 | 3.68 |
| Karnataka | 17.36 | 17.33 | 28.53 | 34.20 | 46.87 | 2.34 |
| Kerala | 37.53 | 39.43 | 42.69 | 44.97 | 66.28 | 3.36 |
| Madhya Pradesh | 23.12 | 25.89 | 46.57 | 44.00 | 52.69 | 2.65 |
| Maharashtra | 40.26 | 57.48 | 45.49 | 53.74 | 63.02 | 1.39 |
| Orissa | 30.55 | 64.17 | 74.25 | 87.93 | 107.24 | 3.13 |
| Rajasthan | 15.71 | 18.24 | 21.67 | 29.03 | 31.10 | 2.51 |
| Tamil Nadu | 299.00 | 303.13 | 299.16 | 293.66 | 369.81 | 5.20 |
| West Bengal | 17.77 | 20.01 | 23.01 | 30.52 | 31.21 | 2.59 |
| All 12 States | 33.35 | 40.30 | 43.00 | 46.18 | 55.89 | 3.56 |
| Constant Prices (1994) |  |  |  |  |  |  |
| Andhra Pradesh | 16.81 | 54.05 | 49.96 | 49.13 | 53.26 | 4.06 |
| Assam | 39.68 | 35.74 | 29.96 | 31.65 | 48.79 | 3.59 |
| Gujarat | 141.66 | 161.84 | 177.80 | 170.59 | 181.38 | 5.01 |
| Haryana | 97.26 | 82.32 | 96.32 | 97.67 | 96.54 | 4.29 |
| Karnataka | 24.86 | 21.56 | 33.20 | 37.42 | 46.87 | 2.83 |
| Kerala | 52.02 | 44.91 | 45.84 | 46.73 | 66.28 | 3.83 |
| Madhya Pradesh | 32.57 | 32.20 | 55.64 | 47.42 | 52.69 | 3.05 |
| Maharashtra | 59.57 | 75.01 | 54.69 | 59.36 | 63.02 | 1.40 |
| Orissa | 44.80 | 81.97 | 86.91 | 95.35 | 107.24 | 3.73 |
| Rajasthan | 20.62 | 19.95 | 22.69 | 27.84 | 31.10 | 2.92 |
| Tamil Nadu | 451.55 | 401.53 | 355.66 | 317.04 | 369.81 | 5.71 |
| West Bengal | 22.44 | 23.34 | 25.86 | 30.98 | 31.21 | 2.97 |
| All 12 States | 50.35 | 53.03 | 52.1 | 50.98 | 55.89 | 4.06 |

*Note*: Expenditure on nutrition includes central and state governments' revenue expenditure on centrally sponsored schemes and state governments' revenue expenditure.

*Source*: Radhakrishna, R., S. Indrakant, and C. Ravi. 1998. India's Integrated Child Development Services Program—Assessment and Options for Reform. Center for Economic and Social Studies. Hyderabad. Processed.